# REVIEWS

"Real . . . raw . . . and very much needed. *Kiss My Curvy Assets* is a great mixture of information, insights, stories, tips, and inspiration written in Lori's sassy and humorous tone, with each chapter packed full of actionable items to help you be your best self. Every woman should read this, if for nothing else than to know she is not alone in the pressure she faces and the insecurities she may have about her body and self-worth." ~ Sally Anderson, CEO Crypto Sally

"This book is a great motivation for all - not only for the ladies! I am curvy as well, struggled all my life, but I am confident with myself (most of the time). I take care of myself, but enjoy food whenever I like . . . yes, I am far beyond perfect! This book gives you a real kick, for your inner 'you.' It is very nice and you can read it more than once, read it by chapter, or flip through it!" ~ Andrea BM, NetGalley

"I love how this book is not here to for all the negative vibes on body image, rather it's about body positivity and embracing what works and feels well for you and your health. It's a book that one can always refer to when they are struggling with body image, self-esteem, self-love and are also considering dieting and healthy eating options. Thank you Netgalley for the eARC because now I know more about 'fad diets' and why people are quickly taken in by them." ~ Dora Archie, NetGalley

"*Kiss My Curvy Assets* will leave you feeling inspired, motivated to kick some self-limiting beliefs, old habits, and patterns to the curb, and take charge of your health because you are forced to examine the quality of your life and health on a holistic level. Lori takes you on a journey of self-love, healing, and empowerment by educating and coaching you every step of the way. Every chapter is filled with fact, humor, a tough yet loving nudge to help you get back to being healthy - on every level. A must read and must-have for every woman!" ~ Tania Moraes-Vaz, Best-selling author, and multi-preneur

"Lori lays out the history of how society pushed women to hate their bodies, judge themselves, and battle for their self-worth. She gives REAL strategies that we can implement to feel more confident and empowered and helps us tell society to kiss off so we can rock our life." ~ Judy Prokopiak, RN, Coach and Life Transition Specialist, Judy Prokopiak Coaching

"A 'take no prisoners' approach to owning our bodies, Lori's message prioritizes health first, not only in our nutrition and exercise - but in the way we nurture our well being and state of mind. It addresses all the insecurities we as women confront daily - and TAKES THEM DOWN!" ~ Samantha Ashley Anderson, Hair Stylist/ Healthy Body Advocate/ Advisor

"Finally, a book that makes sense and appeals to ALL women, regardless of age or fitness experience/knowledge. Lori's approach to health and wellness is refreshing and will no doubt leave you feeling energized. You need to read this book, it's a GAME CHANGER!" ~ Carla-Mellado, Owner/Operator, Mellado Dance Elite

"This book covers two of the most important topics today: body image and self-acceptance. Lori doesn't hold back, keeps it real and authentic. I love the 'R.E.A.L' strategies and 'K.I.S.S Keep it Simple Sexy' principles. Lori's book has the power to change lives. A must read for all women!" ~ Laurie Elizabeth Noh, Nutrition Coach/Owner, Eagle Ridge Fitness

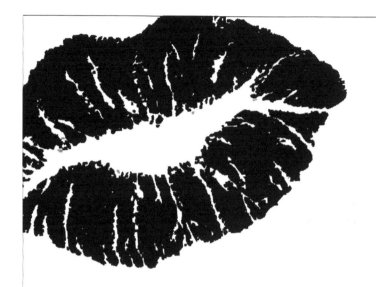

# KISS MY
## *curvy*
## ASSETS

## LORI MORK

KISS MY CURVY ASSETS: EMBRACE, ACCEPT, HIGHLIGHT, AND ROCK THE SHIT OUT OF YOUR BODY!

Published in Canada, for Global Distribution by Golden Brick Road
Publishing House Inc.
www.goldenbrickroad.pub

**FOR MORE INFORMATION EMAIL: LORI@LORIMORK.COM**

ISBN: trade paperback: 978-1-988736-51-8
ebook: 978-1-988736-52-5
Kindle: 978-1-988736-53-2

To order additional copies of this book: orders@gbrph.ca

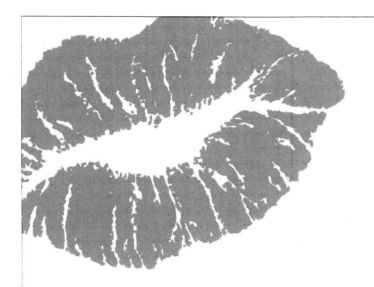

KISS MY
*curvy*
ASSETS

*Dedicated to . . .*

*All the badass babes out there who have felt less than. Babes who have been told they are too skinny or not lean enough, not pretty enough, or not good enough. Babes who have felt pressure to fit some mold, norm, or impossible ideal.*

*YOU FUCKIN' ROCK!*

*This one is for you!*

# CONTENTS

**Introduction**                                                    11

**Chapter 1**
Screw Society and Take Back Control of Your Body Ideals      21

**Chapter 2**
It Takes A Village - Find Your Tribe                         29

**Chapter 3**
Block, Delete, Unfollow, And Rid Yourself Of Social Media Insanity  39

**Chapter 4**
It's What's Inside That Counts - Master Your Mindset         49

**Chapter 5**
Divorce The Scale                                           59

**Chapter 6**
Break Up With Fad Diets                                     69

**Chapter 7**
Stop Giving A Shit About Other People's Opinions —
Just Do You!                                                79

**Chapter 8**
Find Your Four S's - Self-acceptance, Self-love,
Self-esteem, And Self-care                                  89

**Chapter 9**
Achieve The Three M's (Meditation, Mantras, Motivation)     103

**Chapter 10**
Get Naked Frequently - Orgasm Often!                        113

**Chapter 11**
Let Shit Go, Focus On The Future, And Don't Dwell On The Past  123

**Chapter 12**
Abolish The Green-eyed Monster - Jealousy And Comparison  131

**Chapter 13**
Implement Nutrition For Real Life  139

**Chapter 14**
Move Your Assets On Your Own Terms  153

**Chapter 15**
Create Sustainable Goals  165

**Chapter 16**
Check Your H.A.T (Hormones, Adrenals, Thyroid)  173

**Chapter 17**
Wash Your Mouth Out With Soap - Stop With The Swear Words  183

**Chapter 18**
Pave The Way To Better Body Image For Future Women  193

**Chapter 19**
Embrace Your Curves And Assets  203

**Chapter 20**
Get Inspiration From Celebrities
Who Own Their Shape And Body Ideals  213

**Ready To Rock**  227

## INTRODUCTION

For twenty-seven years, I have worked in this crazy fitness industry and have witnessed thousands of women who are broken, upset, sad, depressed, and at their wits' end being so hard on themselves. I have seen countless women with low self-esteem, very little self-worth, and zero self-acceptance. I have watched, and continue to watch, the constant struggle we as women put ourselves through in terms of body ideals and fitness goals. The comparing, the judgements, the self-bullying. Not living our fullest lives and instead keeping up with some rat race that inevitably ends up a hamster wheel, never finding true success. We just keep spinning our wheels in an industry that keeps setting us up to fail. True happiness and success will never be found through diet and exercise alone — there is a bigger picture that everyone is missing. What if there were a way to find true love for our bodies, embrace our shape and curves, and find long-term success with fitness? What if the answer didn't lie in calorie counting or workout routines, but instead with other methods to ensure success from the inside out. What if the keys to our successes have as much to do with the environments we create for ourselves as the sweat, squats, and tread climbing?

We have been brainwashed to believe that when it comes to getting the body we want, it's all about what we are putting in our mouths and the amount of calories we are burning. For decades, we have been programmed to believe this and, like robots, we diet and follow exercise routines. What if I told you there were other tools we could pull out to help us to rock the body we have and ensure sustainable fitness? Twenty chapters in this book, of which only two are about diet and exercise — that leaves eighteen more ways to help you rock the body you have, not just in the short term but for life! This book can help you get there.

Sure, diet and exercise are a part of the process, but in my twenty-seven years in this crazy industry, I have found a little secret that no one has been telling us. The diet industry is a thirty-three billion dollar industry that wants you to think you need those diets and extremes. The secret that this multi-billion-dollar industry doesn't want us to know is it truly goes beyond what we are putting in our mouths and how much we are sweating, and we don't need to sink another dollar into the nonsense and abuse they provide us. It goes so much deeper than the pills, creams, programs, and cults out there in the diet world, so much deeper and more internal. There are many other ways we can embrace our body and finally stop the insanity of not being happy with the skin we are in. We don't need all these tools at once; in fact, we can pick one or two to get started on, and add more as we are ready. Baby steps, chapter by chapter, we can find so many other ways to embrace our bodies, highlight our curves, and rock the shit out of them for a lifetime!

*Kiss my Curvy Assets - Embrace, Accept, Highlight, And Rock The Shit Out Of Your Body!* provides the bigger picture - the complete package. It provides a tool to lean on when we slip back into old habits of negative self-talk, lack of self-acceptance, and the struggle to be healthy or happy with our amazing bodies.

But before we go into these strategies, let's see how we got here. How did the image of the female body evolve to be the monster that we have to live with every day? Let's explore the history and it's changes through the years.[1]

## EVOLUTION OF THE FEMALE BODY IMAGE

**Prehistoric times - 1900s**: For a long time, the focus was on full-figured silhouettes — think Venus, round and pear-shaped bodies, large breasts, all symbolizing fertility. Think Aphrodite, the goddess of sexual love and beauty, who was often portrayed with curves. BA BOOM! Many artists portrayed the "ideal" woman as curvy and voluptuous all the way through to the seventeenth and eighteenth centuries. My kind of peeps! The term used was "Rubenesque," after the painter Rubens, who loved painting plump, rounded, curvy women. Hourglass for days! But to achieve this ideal look, many women needed a corset - a popular undergarment that has made a weird comeback recently and that can cause serious health problems, including internal organ damage, reproductive issues, and even internal bleeding. Corsets were meant to accentuate a woman's curves by cinching in her waist and supporting her bosom, but they did it through pain and suffering, combined with long-term damage. So during this period (specifically what was being promoted by the fashion industry), the ideal body type was curvaceous and voluptuous. Going into the twentieth century, various oil paintings continued to portray women's bodies through plump nudes, but things were slowly taking a turn toward more athletic and slender bodies.

**1900 - 1910s:** During this time period, we saw body images and body ideals labelled "The Gibson girl," a creation of illustrator Charles Dana Gibson. This ideal was portrayed as slender and tall, paired with a giant bust and wide hips. It was a huge exaggeration of the hourglass, achieved by using a corset and pinching the torso and waist significantly.[2]

**1920 - 1950s:** Bring on the eating disorders. In the 1900-1910s, we were already seeing this trend to crazy ratios. Remember the 1920s flapper? Slim, slender bodies appear all over magazines during this period, creating an epidemic of eating disorders. In the 1920s (and also 1980s), the ideal body was the thinnest in all of US history. Tiny little waists and huge breasts became the ideals, but most women were unable to recreate this look and had to resort to extremes like disordered eating to attain it. In the 1940s, we were lucky to see pinup girls and actresses like Marilyn Monroe bring back the fuller body type, but this trend was short-lived. By the 1960s, the images once again became extremely unattainable.

**1960s - 1970s:** One word sums up this era: Twiggy. This fashion icon was everywhere, and so was her impossible body standard set forth to young girls. Although the corset was gone, society was still pressuring

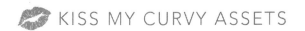 

us to attain this "ideal" body — young and very thin. Now diet and exercise were pushed on us full force. The incidence of severe anorexia nervosa (starving oneself) rose tremendously.

**1970s - 1980s:** Rehabs.com described this era as "Thin is in." Eating disorders and the severe pressure to be thin hit an all-time high, driving people to extreme consequences. Singer Karen Carpenter took her dieting to starvation levels, and the eating disorder eventually claimed her life. This era also saw the rise of the "diet" pills: dangerous amphetamines used to suppress the appetite.

**1980s - 1990s:** Bring on the supermodels! Though images of thin women continued to be mainstream well into the 1980s, these years saw the start of an emphasis on strong, athletic, and toned body types. We had classic supermodels like Cindy Crawford and Naomi Campbell in the 80s. The 90s can be summed up in one word: Baywatch. We all remember busty Pamela Anderson running along the beach with her twenty-inch waist and probably fifty-inch bust. In the 90s, Kate Moss also entered the picture with her skinny body (she was actually nick-named "the waif"). "*Nothing tastes as good as skinny feels,*" Moss was quoted (just *asking* us to have eating disorders in the quest to be skinny and fit the ideal). While eating disorders were at their all-time high, obesity had also crept its ugly head into the picture. Obesity, meaning too much body fat, can increase the risk of health problems including diabetes, heart disease, stroke, arthritis, and even some cancers. So there was this battle of extremes on both sides — the waif vs. the obese. The fashion industry celebrated extreme thinness, while making it seem as though larger bodies were "unhealthy" or "bad." Such intense emotional and psychological pressure on us to fit the ideals and molds.

**2000s:** Insert loss of self-confidence. A review of existing studies on body image and media found that between 1999 and 2006, hospitalizations for eating disorders in the US spiked one hundred and nineteen percent among children under the age of twelve.[3] This younger generation was unable to find their own identities and absorbed so much nonsense from the media and society, all while trying to fit into these ideals and false norms. But it wasn't just eating disorders — now self-confidence was at its lowest, too. Women everywhere were dissatisfied with their bodies and how they looked. Women started to lose their self-love, their self-acceptance.

**2010s to present day:** The rise of social platforms and social media were supposed to bring a new frontier for body-positive expression, but the ideals set forth are still impossible and often faked with filters. These unachievable norms reflect so negatively on our body images and self-worth. While we are making headway in terms of celebrating more curvy and fuller figured women in the media, we still have such a long way to go.

It is crazy to see the evolution of the female curve. Thousands of years ago, sculptures and art showed women's exaggerated curves. Then we hit an era of stick-thin and waif-like models in the magazines. Now it's all about being ripped and lean and taking selfies, and of course the shredded abs and butt pics get the most likes on social media. *Glamour Magazine* found that ninety-seven percent of women are cruel to their bodies every day and are NOT body confident.[4] This makes me both mad and so disappointed that only three percent of us are actually kind to our bodies and rocking them. That is very scary and so incredibly wrong!

This staggering stat doesn't shock me though. As women, we beat ourselves up, compare ourselves to others, and are just evil to our self-worth because we aren't "keeping up." *Will we ever be enough? Will we ever be happy in our own skin? Or will we always strive to look like someone else?* Women, by nature, are supposed to be curvy. Now, some of my non-hourglass friends beg to differ. But the definition of curve is actually not hourglass or full-figured. The definition of curve is to have or take a turn, change, or deviation from a straight line or plane surface without sharp breaks or angularity.[5]

So by that definition, every woman has curves! We aren't flat cardboard boxes! I like to think of our curves, edges, shape, and lines as "assets." Assets are defined as a useful or valuable thing, person, or quality. So why isn't every woman feeling like she can rock her assets!? Each one of us have so much love, valuable qualities, and knowledge to share with the world! And that should be enough. Period.

The "why" of this book came to me when I finally hit a wall. I had witnessed so many women struggling and feeling like they weren't enough. I, myself, was included in this huge mess that society, and now social media, had created. Women everywhere were at a loss for how to find acceptance and love of their bodies and to own their curves and true assets. I knew the time had come to help women shift in the direction of self-acceptance and take back control of our own ideals and self-esteem. I have been in the trenches, and came out alive, but with some permanent scarring. I don't want any more women to suffer like I have.

In a world where we, as women, have been programmed and fed these impossible ideals and images our whole lives, how do we even start the healing? How do we undo the damage? How do we shift our perspective? How do we regain control of how we want to look and feel?

We can find a better way, a better life based on loving the body we have, accepting every curve and edge on it, and highlighting and celebrating our amazing shape! But it takes time, tools, and strategies to change. This book will help you find self-acceptance without crash diets, extremes, yo-yo-ing, low self-worth, and the fitness rat race. There is more to life than the calories you are eating and the fat you are burning. But to get there, we have to address so much more than just the exterior. Let's go on this journey together, with open minds, huge hearts, and a desire to embrace the shit you have and forge ahead to be the best version of yourself — for life. Let's look beyond our eating, beyond our sweat sessions in which we try to sculpt the body, and instead focus on ways to find this self-acceptance, to embrace the body you have, and to highlight it instead of needing to change or transform it. I hope this book will give you all the clarity you desire, to know that *we* define our own body ideals. We are meant to love ourselves, and this includes our body. We need to embrace our curves and shape — and if anyone has a problem with it, *we* have the right to tell them to kiss off.

So what makes me qualified to write this book? What does this girl even know? I want to get going on the important stuff, but first - my story, my *why*.

For three decades of my life, I hated my body, punishing it with every fad and extreme out there. I was so tired of not being able to juggle being a mom and being fit, and I bullied myself when I didn't fit the molds as I saw in society and on social media.

The first time I can remember noticing my body imperfections was around the age of twelve, when I began trying the cabbage soup and grapefruit diets. I can remember that mean boy on the playground calling me "thunder thighs."

My family meant well, but I was born with a naturally fuller body. I was curvy. They used to call me "chunky bum" — I guess they didn't realize that someday, J-lo and Beyonce would make my big booty in style and a must-have or butt implants would be an "in thing!" As far back as I can remember, I have struggled with low self-esteem, feelings of insecurity, dislike for my body, and always desired to be smaller, leaner, better.

Those "thunder thighs" and "chunky bum" comments continued to haunt me and I became obsessive over my imperfections, constantly judging myself. When I got into the fitness industry almost thirty years ago, I put even more pressure on myself to "fit the mold." People expect trainers to have a fit and awesome body. I remember being told, "Nobody wants a *fat* trainer." Your body is your best form of advertising for anyone working in this industry. But what people don't see is the internal damage being caused by the extremes needed to maintain the impossible ideal look. As if it wasn't enough to be abusing myself for all of those years, I decided to dabble in fitness competitions. I was already insanely brutal on myself, so why not allow a panel of judges to pick me apart and send me further into self-hate? This new "hobby" supported my obsession with diet and exercise, and I felt like I fit in with all of the other broken women. I continued to use my weight or pant-size as an indication of my self-worth. I was surrounded by women who never thought they were good enough, bashed themselves constantly, and were always rebounding from harsh dieting methods.

In 2009, I achieved the ultimate goal: I won The Arnold Schwarzenegger Fitness Competition. However, instead of being on a high, I was at my all-time low. Depressed, anxious, not sleeping, barely any energy or zest for life, zero sex drive, hair falling out, and secluding myself socially. I was performing at extremes and was actually being rewarded for clearly having some form of eating disorder. I hit the first of several breaking points and retired from competing, but continued to coach hundreds of women using extreme dieting methods and impossible mental programming.

Then came social media and everything it brings with it. A world that glorifies starvation and crazy overnight fixes with pills and cleanses. A world that constantly presents some "ideal" for us women to strive for. I saw post after post about not having excuses for not being "fit" and "lean." I saw bodies portrayed as something we as women need to punish and abuse in the quest to achieve. As I scrolled through the massive amounts of images slapping me in the face, I continued to see broken women and broken methods. I saw a society that was expecting us to fit some impossible mold.

In 2010, I decided to shift my focus and instead of helping women be "fit," I would coach them in holistic wellness. I decided my main goal was to help women achieve wellness in all aspects of their life and think longer term and sustainable, over short-term and damaged.

# INTRODUCTION

Over the past nine years, I have worked with thousands of women who all seem to experience the same concerns. "I want to reach my fitness goals, but I am very broken inside. I am scared, confused by all that is out there, and torturing myself with impossible fads, magic pills, drinks, cleanses, and extreme programming. Nothing is working and I feel like I'm drowning." I made it my mission, my movement, to help as many women as possible get out of this dark, sad, deep hole that the diet industry was holding us hostage in. I needed to reach out to women everywhere, to help them change the way they viewed themselves and the norms that were created for us, to scream out loud and reclaim control of our bodies. I was angry, a little hostile (I'm a Scorpio, so very hostile), and guilty that I had contributed to this insanity for decades, and I was ready to make a change and finally help other women escape the madness. From my breakdown, I found my breakthrough, and my hope for you is that, by reading this book, you will find the answers you are looking for as well, the help you need to forge ahead and be the best version of yourself.

I hope this book can assist you in feeling better about your body and undo some of the damage and internal chaos the dieting world may have caused you. I want you to finally find the way to embracing your body and finding sustainable fitness. In twenty chapters, I'll give you twenty ways to get there. Not all of them are needed. Taking it day by day, chapter by chapter, we can forge ahead together to create this movement of embracing, accepting, highlighting, and rocking the shit out of our amazing bodies.

*I keep telling myself that I'm a human being who's not made to look like a doll, and that who I am as a person is more important then whether at the moment I have a nice figure.*

~ EMMA WATSON

## ROCK WITH US

Join our tribe! You do not have to face changes and challenges alone. Success relies heavily on community, and as you're reading through the book and being inspired, learning (or just plain old have questions), reach out and let us know. It's so much easier to accomplish change when you surround yourself with people who are on the same page - so, let's hold each other accountable and make it a party!

At the end of each chapter you'll find an invitation to share your thoughts, ideas, and pics to #kissmycurvyassets. The more you share, the more we all benefit!

If you're a bit more private, this space can also be used for you to record your favorite parts of the chapter, write some kick-ass self-reflection, top tips/take-aways or good, old-fashioned reminders to yourself.

Just look for the box with the ROCK WITH US heading at the very end of each chapter.

You'll also see that we've added some space for notes and thoughts- a place where you can make this book, and the changes you're inspired to make, your own. Pens are analog, I know, but sometimes just putting a thought on paper can help you transform it into something more concrete and more real. AND it lets us see a little bit more about you if you take a pic and share.

So who is ready to rock the shit out of their assets with me?!

## NOTES

_____

_____

_____

# CHAPTER 1

# SCREW SOCIETY AND TAKE BACK CONTROL OF YOUR BODY IDEALS

*You define beauty for yourself. Society doesn't define your beauty.*

~ LADY GAGA

Ah, my youth. As I sit on my patio thinking about all the great television shows I grew up with and how they contributed to my amazing body image . . . wait, I had a terrible body image . . .

Let's reflect. I am a 70s and 80s wild child, so if you are with me in your forties and fifties, you may remember all the amazing different shapes and sizes that the most popular TV shows portrayed. *Charlie's Angels* had tons of different-sized women . . . wait . . . errr . . . who was the curvy, chunky angel again? There wasn't one! Okay, what about *Three's Company* . . . hmmm . . . Janet and Chrissy Snow surely weren't more than a size zero! *Dukes of Hazzard* had to have a more realistic body image . . . oh goodness, no thunder thighs are fitting into those Daisy Duke jean cut-offs. *Dallas, Dynasty, Happy Days* all had more small frames and minimal body fat with zero muscle.

Okay, our era failed epically, but the 90s had to have gotten better, right? Shows like *Friends, Saved By The Bell, Dawson's Creek* must have presented more fuller figured or realistic bodies . . . Whoops, epic fail yet again. *Beverly Hills 90210* and *Melrose Place* were . . . also not filled with anything but skinny, small, and smaller. Well, thankfully as children, we were surrounded by epic roles models of insane shapes and different sizes — just look at the Disney princesses . . . oh no! Not one of them has quad muscles, not one of them has a bigger frame, and for sure, not one of them has athletic or fuller arms.

Throughout our youth, we were conditioned to believe in the "one-size-fits-all-body." And present day media hasn't changed much either - everywhere we turn, we are bombarded with pictures of the ideal body. All across various media platforms — television, magazines, billboards, and websites — we see celebrities, fashion models, talk show hosts, and others in the public eye cast as role models for what it means to be successful and popular. Their body weight, appearance, and beauty are often associated with their popularity and wealth. The media holds our minds captive as it exercises a tight rein over our self-worth and our self-esteem. Television, internet, movies, and the media have a strong grip on women's personal perceptions of what beauty or fitness is supposed to look like. As women, we are bombarded with a barrage of literal and subliminal messaging from every direction telling us what we should look like, what we should eat, and who we should aspire to be. These images and ideals contribute to negative body image, low self-confidence, preoccupation with diet, leaving us to feel as though our bodies are inadequate. We start thinking, feeling, and behaving as though we are not enough.

Because of this, our egos and esteem are at an all-time low, and eating disorders at an all-time high. By the age of seven, one in four children will have engaged in some sort of dieting behaviors. Between 1999 and 2006, eating disorders in the US had spiked one hundred and nineteen percent in children aged twelve and under.[6] GASP! Neuroscience has shown that whatever you focus on shapes your brain. If you are constantly thinking negative thoughts about your body, that neural pathway becomes stronger - and those thoughts become habits. Wow, that is a little brainy and deep - in layman's terms, your brain is telling you to "stop thinking bad shit about yourself or it will convince you it's true." Believe that you aren't worthy, and you won't feel worthy. Bit by bit, we slide down the rabbit-hole of comparison, feeling negative about ourselves. These self-loathing feelings are further magnified when we see others fall into the same trap of negative thinking.

Even though society can be a major culprit in influencing our thoughts and lives, we must take ownership for playing into the unrealistic expectations and ideals set by society. Our modus operandi is to bully ourselves with negative self-talk. Think about it: Whenever we are having a bad day, we take it out on our body with insults. We turn into the inner "mean girl." Why? This behavior and inner dialogue is imbibed from such a young age and as we grow older, we continue to carry it with us without paying any attention to its long-term impact on our lives.[7]

I found this great letter written by Claire Foster,[8] and it really does sum up the damage caused by the unrealistic ideals that society holds us women to:

*"To the media: You may not know me, but oh I know you. I know the monster you've placed inside of us. I see the unrealistic standards you set for our beauty and the underlying demons that accompany it. The eating disorders and radical dieting fads. Lose 10 pounds in 5 days. Look 25 forever. Hounding us. Hurting us. When we were children, we would look in the mirror and see ourselves how we truly were: human and healthy. From all fronts, we are now told that this unattainable image is beautiful. Women around the world are starving themselves, injecting their bodies with toxic chemicals to match this photo edited and plastic model of the female form. They say a picture speaks a thousand words; well it's clear what your pictures say: Unattainable. Unhealthy. But it doesn't have to be this way, not if I can help it. It is more beautiful to be healthy and to nourish your body than to conform to a cosmetically engineered, photoshopped magazine cover. Instead of comparing stomachs, compare the positive things you do for your body. Be kind to your body, nourish your soul. You'd be amazed what happens when you stop beating yourself up. I know I am. Media, you may not know me, but I sure as hell know you and I think it's time to show you the door. From, Claire Foster."*

In the introduction, I showed how the societal expectation of the ideal female body image has evolved over time and has influenced how we as women feel about ourselves and what we aspire to be. The ever-evolving and unrealistic female body image ideals keep getting harder and harder for us real women to achieve. To see true long-term fitness success and to find the body we have always been striving for, we need to dig deeper and map out *our* true body ideals. We need to tune into what will make us feel good, feel loved, and feel fierce about our body, from the inside out. I'm talking here about *your* ideals — what is right for your body, not what someone else tells you to aspire to, not society and its insane standards and norms.

What does the term "body ideals" even mean? Body ideals are defined as the body type that is regarded as most suitable and attractive for a person, considering one's age, gender, build, and culture.[9] So by that definition, we need to take away anything we have learned in the media. Take away that very first toy you probably had (Barbie - whose measurements and body pertain to only one in every one hundred thousand American women, usually due to some type of life-threatening condition). Throw out those magazines with models who are beyond thin and all those other media images that represent a shape and physique that many of us should not and could not achieve.

So now what? How can we remove those images and discover what we truly find attractive? Pretend you have a clean slate and can choose whatever you like. Choose your body based on your real life, your physical demands, and your genetics. Sit back and ask yourself two questions:

**1. Am I healthy?**

**2. Does my body allow me to do the things I want in life?**

If you answered yes to those two questions, then your body is already ideal. There is nothing wrong with wanting to enhance or highlight what you already have, but striving to look like the images presented in the media is a slippery slope. The body doesn't like to be forced into anything! So when we impose these unrealistic ideals, the body will fight back psychosomatically. Impossible diets make you feel disconnected from your family and friends, as you become busy with obsessing and overtraining. Your children witness this unhealthy relationship with food and your body and internalize it subliminally - planting the seed of body-shaming and self-loathing in the next generation of young girls.

But being skinnier, smaller, prettier, younger, leaner does not make us more worthy or better. For example, I am a taller woman (five feet and eight inches tall) and I have stronger, fuller legs. Strong enough to run around after my kids, strong enough to climb steep hills walking with my dog, and strong enough to lift heavy weights at the gym. I don't mind these thicker thighs, and I would keep them on my ideal body. I was born with an hourglass figure, and I naturally like the smaller waist-to-hip ratio.

Thankfully, my own genetics support it. I feel like the smaller waist and the big old round booty and wide hips is an ideal look for me. I enjoy continuing to round out the hourglass by using my weight training programs to focus on building wider shoulders and a tighter, rounder booty. I also don't enjoy when my face is depleted and sunken in from being too thin, so I am naturally pulled toward a full-figured physique. Done! Sign me up!

But remember, these are *my* ideals.

You need to have *your* own ideals, based on your genetics, your life, and your desires. Remember those two questions again: Are you healthy? Does your body allow you to do the things you want to do in life? At the end of the day, the only thing you can work on is becoming the best version of yourself.

So how can we fight this thirty-three-billion-dollar industry that continues to invent newer, impossible body image ideals and that perpetuates this cycle of self-hate? How do we take back our power? We do this by accepting the images at face value and acknowledging that they are graphically enhanced, fake, photoshopped, and unrealistic. We do this by refusing to accept them as the norm or ideal. Instead, we focus on our strengths and accomplishments, repeat affirmations and mantras, and collectively start a movement to ensure that these ideals are changed and that honest images and messages are portrayed. As women, we need to come together — fierce, empowered, and aware — to ensure that change does take place, no matter how big or small, so that we can stop being true to the false ideals we are surrounded with and start being true to ourselves and to what makes us feel good.

I came up with an easy way to tune into your wants and needs for your ideal body and body image. It involves reframing and redefining what is real or, in this case, R.E.A.L:

| R | **REALITY** | Is the image you are viewing real or even realistic? |
|---|---|---|
| E | **ESTEEM** | Is the image you are keeping as your ideal helping your self-esteem, or stripping it down? |
| A | **ACCEPTANCE** | There is no perfect! Aim to accept and highlight what could be perceived as "flaws," and turn them into your strengths. |
| L | **LOVE** | At the end of the day, nothing matters if you don't show yourself and your body love. If you find a place of love for yourself, that is when you control how you feel. |

So what now? Well, once we take back control of our own body ideals, we can stand strong together as women and lobby for body positivity around the world. The hair and skin care company, Dove, embarked on its own body positivity campaign, *Campaign For Real Beauty,* in 2004 with a series of viral advertisements portraying the differences between women as they're depicted in ads and women's actual appearance without any makeup or digital enhancement. Dove's print ads have also shown women of various weights, shapes, and sizes, without alteration. Additionally, many celebrities have also taken control to ensure that they own the shape and curves of their bodies in order to be a role model for those watching them. In a later chapter, we will go into detail on some of these amazing celebs who rock the shit out of their bodies!

At the beginning of this chapter, we saw how we have been fed these images and almost pre-programmed to believe *this* is how we should look, *this* is what we are supposed to aspire to. So what will happen when we take back control of our own ideals? We will feel fierce, loved, confident, and more at home in our own skin, in our own body. No longer will we feel the pressure to conform to the ideals dictated by society, because we will know that we are more than enough and that we are beautiful in our own right. We have the blueprint of the R.E.A.L self body image - Reality, Esteem, Acceptance, and Love. Once we adopt these principles into our lives, we can take that huge leap forward to find our long-term health and fitness goals, on *our* own terms, free from any negative feelings to ourselves or unrealistic expectations of ourselves. So move over, *Charlie's Angels* — we are ready to be our own new angel, and rock the shit out of our bodies!

*I really don't care what I look like that much. I think women out there should just be happy with the way they look. They shouldn't really try to conform to any kind of stereotype. Just be happy and hopefully healthy.*

~ REBEL WILSON

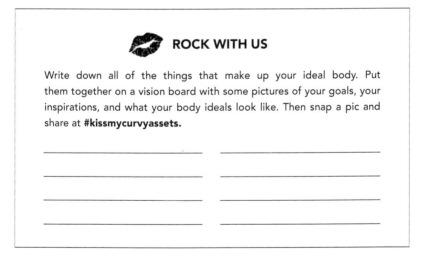

**ROCK WITH US**

Write down all of the things that make up your ideal body. Put them together on a vision board with some pictures of your goals, your inspirations, and what your body ideals look like. Then snap a pic and share at **#kissmycurvyassets**.

# CHAPTER 2

# IT TAKES A VILLAGE - FIND YOUR TRIBE

*I don't know what I would have done so many times in my life if I hadn't had my girlfriends.*

~ REESE WITHERSPOON

Tribe, clan, group, community, posse, girl-squad, team, gang, network — no matter what you decide to call it, you need that solid foundation of women around you to help you continue owning your shit. As women, we rise, dominate, and succeed when we bond together and band together, encouraging one another, empowering each other, and celebrating one another. There is strength in numbers; the power of a group of women is phenomenal. Think of the power of tribes of women all over the world embracing, accepting, and helping each other own their true essence and power to create their ultimate body ideals on their own terms. Without societal pressures or social media nonsense. Without pressure to be a part of a mold that does not work for us. Without feeling like we aren't enough. Think of how it feels to be struggling, doing the same thing day in and day out, trying to find your way, only to feel like you are in a never-ending maze — until you come across a group of people who reach out and extend a helping hand to help you dig yourself out the depths of self-destruction.

As humans, we were built to be social creatures. We are designed to crave and operate with a sense of community and tribe. This basic need for tribe and connection has not changed in modern times. No matter how digitally advanced we are as a society, we all want to feel like we belong, we all want that human connection and a powerful sense of community. Going at it alone is no fun, nor is it the way to live your life. Imagine how beautiful, calming, encouraging, and exciting it would be to surround yourself with like-minded women, speaking the same language, forging ahead together with the same values. Imagine having a sisterhood where you can share your journey, support one another, work together, and develop strong, empowering personal relationships with each other.

I wanted to find my tribe, but I struggled for so long. You see, the fitness industry pretends to be body-positive, putting on a mask of self-acceptance and love, only to show their true colors once you're signed on. Everywhere I turned, I saw women pretending they had self-acceptance, yet they were so messed up and still trying to live up to the illusions encouraged by social media. If anything, their social media posts of their abs, butts, and thighs were simply feeding into their toxic thought pattern.

So instead of searching any further for my tribe, I decided to create my own. I decided to write this book and hopefully reach out to every woman who may be experiencing this exact struggle so they can feel welcomed into my tribe, or become empowered to create and lead their own. Think of your tribe as links on a chain — one link is amazing, but a series of links locked together makes for a strong chain. The more I began to reach out, the more I came across women who felt the same — women who had a vision, a strong and empowering voice to share, and a collaborative and nurturing spirit to join me on this journey.

As women, we are powerful together. We can change the way we view ourselves by abolishing societal ideals and norms, and replacing them with our own version of what works for us. Although I do have Facebook groups set up, you don't have to wait for me — you can seek out your own tribe. Heck, start your own posse and co-lead this movement with me!

So how do we go about looking for a suitable fem-powered girl-squad? Much like being the new kid in school, it can be scary, over-whelming, and confusing. Additionally, it can be laced with completely insincere individuals whom we will have to sift through to find our genuine, soul-connected tribe.

Here are some tips on how to find your ideal tribe and maintain that connection:

**Remember your WHY.** Why are you looking for this support? Why are you doing this? Why is it important to you to make a change?

**Be aware of what it is that you need from your tribe and what you are looking for in a tribe.** Tough love peeps, mama bears to coddle, or besties to laugh with. What is it that you need most to help you on your journey?

**Leave your judgments in a trashcan. Everyone has their own journey, respect that.** Seriously, I know it is easy for our minds to go down the judgment route instantly, but remember that these women might need you a bit more than you need them. What I mean by this is that it's okay to find women who aren't as far along in their journey to self-acceptance — maybe you can pave the way to guide them on their path.

**Surround yourself with like-minded people who LIVE their talk.** Remember, social media is filled with people saying the buzzwords, talking the talk, and then turning around and not really walking the walk. Surround yourself with those who take messy but brave action, and you too, will start living an empowered life. One big or small action at a time.

**Be brave. Put yourself out there.** Ask others to connect. Start an inspirational social media page that shows your journey to self-love and body acceptance. The more we put ourselves out there, the more other women can see the true change that can come, the genuine internal transformations, and lose the pressure to be "perfect."

**Stay true to your values and avoid getting sucked into the rabbit hole of negativity again.** Consciously choosing to stay aligned with our values takes effort, but practice makes perfect. There will be some moments when it might feel easier to slip back into old ways instead of consciously reframing our inner and outer dialogue. Ensure that your tribe is there to lift you up instead of enabling negative thought patterns, negative self-talk, and old habits.

I have a client who came to me at her absolute rock bottom moment. You see, she had jumped from diet to diet, fad to fad, extreme to extreme. She thought she had finally found her posse. She joined this "challenge" that used all of the buzzwords, like healthy, long-term, not extreme, sustainable. She invested her money and was so pumped to be on her way. Except it didn't go the way she imagined it would. Like a wolf disguised in sheep's clothing, their true colors were revealed about three weeks in when the tribe leader began pitching a top multi-level marketing (MLM) product that was a dieting extreme. She kept pushing this product onto all the group members, insisting that they sell it and try to get others to do the same. There was nothing new, empowering, or refreshing about the mindset. This tribe had an icky tone about it, thanks to the leader — its intentions were not genuine and didn't come from a place of service or support.

And *this* is that vicious cycle I keep talking about. The health, wellness, and fitness industry is a multi-billion-dollar industry, and for every two individuals who want to earn an income and make a heartfelt impact, there will always be another two or more people who don't really care about serving anyone else but themselves — they only care about the dolla dolla bills, y'all, and their fifteen minutes of fame.

My client had been on an emotional roller coaster of insincere and toxic sisterhood. The hopes and dreams she had of finally finding the support she needed were crushed. So much for finding a tribe, right? She could have quit trying and just accepted that she would never find her way or her tribe; she could have just settled for less than what she truly deserved. But she didn't stop looking. She found me, and together we worked to help her rediscover her self-worth, self-love, and genuine appreciation for her body. She doesn't even look back on the past, since that is so far behind her. She has a new tribe, a new outlook, and a new body to match (really, just the same amazing body she always had, except now, she sees it, appreciates it, and celebrates it!)

"Find your tribe!" "Join a sisterhood!" "Discover your soul clan!" All of this sounds so easy-peasy, but in reality, it can be challenging to implement. Period. *Mic drop.* But how do we even go about seeking out women who are on the same journey as us? Where can we find them?

**The gym.** You are at the gym working out and enhancing your body; that gym is filled with other women on the same journey. Once you dig through the meat market of sweaty men, you will see that quiet woman in the corner of the ladies-only section who is looking just as lost as you once were. She makes no eye contact and is just trying to work out and enhance her body like the rest of us. Maybe it's time to stop hiding behind the lens of self-focus and solo workouts and look around to connect with like-minded women — if not as a workout partner, then in a group class. The best place to truly connect with other women at the gym is in a fitness class. It's already more of a sense of community. I have been a group fitness instructor for twenty-seven years, and I can say that I have connected with more women on a deeper level than I could have imagined. You come together in a smaller room, say, a spin class. You laugh, sing to the music, and move your bodies together. There is usually time to connect before and after class, and even beyond the spin class bike. I see so many women leave my classes to grab some coffee or a bite to eat, only to later attend each other's baby showers and create lasting, life-long friendships.

**Not into the gym or fitness classes? Then team sports are another fun way to meet your tribe.** Soccer, baseball, volleyball, hockey, a local running club, rock climbing — the list is endless. You are bound to meet at least one person on the same journey as you.

**The office.** Whoever said you cannot find office besties didn't know what they were talking about! No matter where you work, there might be some women who are looking for a community in this whole embrace-your-body movement. I have a client who reached out to five other women at her workplace and they created their own little "fitness community." They would go for walks together at lunch, meet every morning for workouts at the office gym, and even bring potlucks of wicked recipes to share with each other to help one another achieve their fitness goals. They would even partake in little challenges, such as squat challenges in which they would all perform fifty squats at their desk. Another client once had a group of twelve women at work who would send each other motivational emails just to help them keep pushing forward toward their fitness goals. They took their own "before" pics and did a fun photoshoot at the end to show their "after" results. Never underestimate what a group of supportive women who hold you accountable to walk your talk can do for your and the quality of your life.

**Turn your frenemy, aka social media, into your new BFF / connection powertool!** I say this because social media can be a double-edged sword of positivity and negativity. Sift through the superficial chaos and negativity to discover people whose accounts inspire you and move you to be more authentic in your life. Never underestimate the power of following the right people on social media and listening to podcasts. Use your intuition and find those who truly resonate with you. I have found some amazing soul sisters on the internet — we lift each other up, inspire and support one another no matter where we are at in our journey. Reach out to someone who posts things that impact you or truly move your heart and stimulate your mind. You will be shocked that these truly real women will connect back. Your comment on their post or direct message to them might even be just what they needed to boost their esteem and confidence.

**Women's networking events are the -ish!** So, here's a wayback playback — when I was in my twenties, I actually sold real estate. And boy, was I good at it, all because I was the networking queen! I joined breakfast groups and business luncheons, I went to every wine social night in the city. I worked the room by being myself and letting my passion speak for itself. I knew everyone's name, and if someone new joined our events, I would be the first to go up to them and make them feel welcome. The connections I made by simply showing up genuinely and being present in those moments were insane! In turn, I was top in my

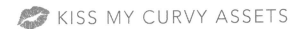 

office because you better believe that anyone I connected with usually thought of me and my real estate services whenever they were buying or selling a house. You don't have to be self-employed or have a big business to attend these networking events. There are so many groups of women that come together, have special speakers or presenters on a variety of great topics, and find time to connect with others. It's amazing to see what can be possible if you take the first step by showing up and putting yourself out there. You will most definitely attract individuals who have the same mindset, values, and goals.

**Got kids? Mom groups rule!** You are not alone, Mama. Remember when you had a baby and there were all these neighborhood mom groups that would meet to "Strollercize" or just hang out? This wasn't for the babies — this was for the mamas. It's easy to feel alone, isolated, and lost when you have a baby, because your life primarily revolves around caring for your new bundle of joy. I remember feeling like I lost myself. I didn't recognize myself, there was no sense of normalcy anymore; I felt so lonely in this newest marathon called motherhood. Knee deep in baby poo and sleepless nights, I was on the verge of having a breakdown. Then I took my tired-ass body into that first mama group meeting, and actually connected with other women who were in crazy-town just like I was. I remember feeling relieved to know that other mums could relate to how I felt. It felt so good to laugh, cry, and talk about literally everything with other women who were going through the same nonsense. Fitness and body goals are no different. In these groups, you can connect with others who are also on the journey to find their bodies again.

**Craigslist (don't knock it yet!).** I know, it sounds a little desperate, but websites such as Craigslist can actually be great to start your own little tribe. Putting yourself out there and searching for others with the same issues, interests, or direction as you can form a really successful posse. Now be smart here, folks. There are a lot of creepers out there, so when you initially meet, don't be all *Criminal Minds* or *Law and Order Special Victims Unit* and be meeting up in dark alleys at midnight. Instead, pick a really busy and public place to have your initial meeting. I had a client who used Craigslist to find others who wanted to hike. She was able to find a dozen women who loved hiking and were looking for others to experience some of the finest hikes out there. They would also have movie and wine nights and found that they had many other things in common in addition to hiking.

**Take a cooking class — a healthy one!** I have a client who eats "mostly" vegan. When she was transitioning to mostly plant-based, she was at a loss for some good recipes and was sick of having spinach salads and acai bowls. She enrolled in a wicked eight-week cooking class and got some killer vegan recipes. She also met some kick-ass people in this program, and they ended up hitting yoga classes together, going on bike rides, and even having potluck nights when they could try out the recipes they had learned. Like-minded people connecting over healthy, nutritious, and delicious food — who knew!

**Get a dog.** Yes, good old Fido is an amazing way to connect with those around you. I have met some amazing peeps just from walking my dogs! I was once at the local dog park (I have a Goldendoodle, Sadie, who is four-years-old, and a Labradoodle, Sam, who is four months), and although I had seen this one woman with her dog there many times, I never knew her as anyone other than "Cosmo's owner." One day, she actually started up a conversation with me about fitness. She complimented me on my arms and told about her weekly workout plan and how she was doing a Crossfit competition. We connected, exchanged numbers, and ended up meeting to walk the dogs together. You best believe I was there cheering her on at at her Crossfit competition, and although it's not my cup of tea, I was so inspired by how fit and strong everyone was out there.

Fitness and finding self-acceptance can be a struggle. It's like an addiction, and just like most addictions, you have (and need) a support network. Like Alcoholics Anonymous (AA), you have weekly meetups to support each other, ensure accountability, share daily wins and struggles, and truly connect with others who just as committed to bettering themselves. Fitness should be no different. We shouldn't need to go it alone when trying to embrace our bodies. Having a sponsor, or a mentor, or a supportive community is a big way to help ensure long-term success. We all fall back into old mindset beliefs, thought patterns, negative self-talk, and bad habits. But with the help of a supportive tribe or community, we have that shoulder to lean on, that voice of reason, and the accountability we need. As a result, not only will we embrace our body, but we will continue to rock the shit out of it and reach those fitness goals for the long run.

*One friend with whom you have a lot in common is better than three with whom you struggle to find things to talk about.*

~ MINDY KALING

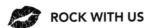

**ROCK WITH US**

Grab a piece of paper and set up 2 columns. On one side, list all of the people in your squad. On the other side, list the most amazing thing about each of them. Take a pic and share it with our community at **#kissmycurvyassets**. Remember, there is strength in numbers when women rock the shit out of their bodies together.

# CHAPTER 3

# BLOCK, DELETE, UNFOLLOW, AND RID YOURSELF OF SOCIAL MEDIA INSANITY

*Now every girl is expected to have Caucasian blue eyes, full Spanish lips, a classic button nose, hairless Asian skin with a California tan, a Jamaican dance hall ass, long Swedish legs, small Japanese feet, the abs of a lesbian gym owner, the hips of a nine year old boy, the arms of Michelle Obama, and doll tits . . . the person closest to actually achieving this look is Kim Kardashian, who, as we all know, was made by Russian scientists to sabotage our athletes. Everyone else is struggling.*

~ TINA FEY

Today is a day filled with promise, and I am ready to take it head on. As I eat my breakfast, I decide to open my phone and scroll through my Facebook newsfeed — only to view posts galore showcasing ripped abs, tight glutes, and constant body "perfection." I quickly run back to change my outfit, since it makes me look even fatter than I am; instead, I opt for the muumuu to hide my fat butt.

While grabbing my favorite coffee at Starbucks en route to work, I scroll through my Instagram feed, only to see fitness model after fitness model telling me about the latest "skinny tea" or "waist trainer" I absolutely must have or bouncing through how-to-lunge videos barking, "No excuses, you need to do like I do and be like me." I decide to toss the muffin I just purchased, since my stomach rolls do not need to grow any further.

The grand finale of the day - feeling disgusted with the way I look, I decide to skip lunch and dinner. After work, I relax on my big old sofa with my laptop and peruse different videos on Youtube, only to see ad after ad of happy, thin models giving me a play-by-play while they blend up smoothies and tell me how to get a bikini body in ten days. *Wow, my life must suck because I am not thin like them.* I decide that I surely need to hit the gym "die-hard" for at least three hours, but instead, I end up drinking a bottle of wine, gorging myself in despair on a plate of nachos, and crawling into bed loathing my appearance. You're now surrounding yourself with your positive, kickass tribe of women warriors. So why on earth are you letting some inauthentic internet influencer damage your self esteem?

A lot of us do this little dance with the modern-day devil-in-disguise, otherwise known as social media. Do you remember the first time you felt hurt, upset, beaten down, or caught in the trap of the social media comparisonitis? As if it wasn't enough to have society pushing unrealistic images on us, let's throw in the insanity of social media platforms. We begin our day feeling good about ourselves, only to be stripped down by the images we constantly see on Facebook, Instagram, Youtube, Snapchat, Twitter, and many more to come. When used effectively, with purposeful and aligned intention coupled with real, raw, honest vulnerability, social media can be a magical and inspiring tool. However, with the pressure to be perfect and fit into unrealistic ideals, it has now turned into a loud den of lies, filters (#nofilter but ya know, there is still a filter applied), body-positive yet body-shaming space, spreading scars and utter chaos over our self-esteem and confidence. With "fitspo" hitting all of the hashtags (does anyone remember life before we knew what a hashtag was?), women are supposed to encourage health, fitness, and community. In reality, though, we end up with a collection of images showcasing results that may be impossible to obtain without resorting to extremes.

I call #completebullshit.

Social media is loaded with images, unrealistic ideals, and insane stereotypes that aim to influence us and drive us into this comparison game. Social media is failing us and keeping us feeling like failures by trapping us in a sea of self-criticism. We compare ourselves to what we see and then look in the mirror and feel we will never be good enough. We continue to struggle with accepting our bodies for what they are. This striving for constant self-improvement is getting old and tiring, and it can turn into an unhealthy obsession. In the past, we could ignore the impossible ideals set out for us by not turning on the television, or not buying the magazines. But now, it is almost second nature for us to reach for our phone and open a social media app. These images are everywhere! It's impossible to hide from them. Here is the big secret. These social media selfies are people's highlight reels. To get those perfectly ripped abs shot, they often take ten to twelve photos, use Photoshop and proper lighting, and of course never post their period-bloated bellies!

As I was researching social media and the impact it has on us, I came across this description from Rachel Simmons:

*The meteoric rise of the 'wellness' industry online has launched an entire industry of fitness celebrities on social media. Millions of followers embrace their regimens for diet and exercise, but increasingly, the drive for 'wellness' and 'clean eating' has become stealthy cover for more dieting and deprivation. This year, an analysis of fifty so-called 'fitspiration' websites revealed messaging that was indistinguishable, at times, from pro-anorexia (pro-ana) or 'thinspiration' websites. Both contained strong language inducing guilt about weight or the body, and promoted dieting, restraint, and fat and weight stigmatization.*[10]

Sadly, we can't "unfollow" everyone. We truly would be blocking and unfollowing the majority of posts if we didn't want to see the abs, booty, or body shots. I have tried deleting my social media accounts four times. Yes, I have completely left this insane world four times, only to be enticed back in by the fact I never heard from anyone unless I read their status on Facebook. So how can we change our perception of ourselves and what we see on social media? Is it possible for us to become more intentional and selective about what we allow into our news feeds? Like I said earlier, social media can be a great outlet and resource when used with purpose. It's not all bad — there is some good information out there. We can find some delicious recipes, motivational posts, and inspiring stories. We can dig through all of the ass shots taken by dirty bathroom mirrors and find posts that impact us in a more positive way. I want you to try this the next time you are scrolling and liking. Whenever you engage in a post that brings up those feelings of comparison, self-criticism, or "not good enough," remind yourself: *These people are not me. It's okay if I don't match them perfectly, the world is filled with many different bodies in many different shapes and size. That is their real life — I have my own!*

When talking about social media insanity, I have to bring up the #noexcuses story. I see this hashtag and comment a lot. Some hot little twenty-two-year-old blonde in a super tight bra top, booty shorts, spray tan, hair extensions, and full make-up tells her "followers" that there are "no excuses." You should all have the body you want, you should all look like her, it's easy, and there are NO EXCUSES for not being ripped and lean. Instead of #noexcuses, I call #bullshit.

There are plenty of excuses — sorry, let's reframe that. There are plenty of *reasons* why your fitness regimen has suffered and been put on the back burner. I get it — different life stages will demand different levels of attention, leaving you with little to no time to stick to your fitness routine. The difference between letting these "excuses" rule your life and prioritizing your own health and wellbeing lies in finding what works for you and establishing your own version of what staying fit or healthy looks like. For some of you, this might mean being active for twenty minutes every day. Meanwhile, someone else may be happy if they managed to get to a group class at least twice a week, ate healthy meals every day, and got some relaxation.

Back to the reasons someone might not have fitness as their top priority. My own personal first two reasons for lacking in the fitness department involve me being a *mom* to my children, Brooklyn and Beckham, who are now twelve and sixteen-years-old. One child needs to be chauffeured all over town, while the other cannot make his own sandwich or get his own fruit (maybe because I was bit of a helicopter mom). Trying to keep a little human being alive means that sometimes your workout doesn't happen, even if it was scheduled in your calendar.

I have another reason called *bills*, which means sometimes I need to work instead of hitting the gym.

I have a third reason called *aging*. I am forty-three-years-old and have been in perimenopause since I was thirty-four, so sometimes my hormones get all messed up and I gain weight or sometimes my energy isn't the same as when I was a spunky twenty-year-old.

Finally, I have this last reason called, "I don't care as much about always being shredded with a six-pack and tight glutes; I found a balance that works for my real life. I like wine, I enjoy it with friends, and my life doesn't allow me to always focus on how my body looks."

That is me. That is my life. I constantly hit social media and see that twenty-two-year-old blonde girl lunging her heart out and screaming NO EXCUSES. Videoing herself doing lunges and being shredded might be real life for her; she's probably single with no children, and her only job might be to video herself on Instagram and hope for fame. That might be her actual life plan, but you might be in the same boat as me and clearly thinking that this is not the case for you. Everyone has their own circumstances that they need to juggle in their daily lives. Your *real* life also changes, and what works for you now in this present moment might not work when you birth a second baby or change jobs. The concept of time also changes as your life evolves - perhaps you are someone who had some time to yourself in the past, but that seems to have changed due to family circumstances, such as divorce or illness.

The problem with social media is that it ignores these multiple priorities and instead subliminally controls how we feel about our body ideals. It also chips away at our self-esteem by making us feel or think that we aren't good enough, we do not work hard enough, we are not lean enough, or we are not enough, period - recall, comparisonitis. Why does social media get to dictate what our ideal body looks and feels like? Why do these little posts hold so much power over our thoughts, our emotions, and how we perceive ourselves and our success? Do those posting this nonsense know what women struggle with on a daily basis? Are they aware that our body is just the vessel that moves our soul around?

Just like we can take back the reins from society and push for more body positivity, we need to bring the same awareness to social media. We do this by choosing who we follow and which posts we engage in - be it likes or comments, and by knowing when to turn off the devices, and turn up for a session with your peeps.

Can we just look, acknowledge, and not allow these images to become internalized for us? Instead of looking to social media to find roles models. Let's be our own fucking role models. Let's set our own standard for body ideals, and then find programming that supports *our* real life (not the highlight reel) and our fitness goals. Let's stand strong together and stop allowing these images and posts to tear down our self-worth. Heck, let's start posting more inspiring posts, lifting other women up instead of assuming we know what they are going through or what their struggles are. Just because someone doesn't work out as hard as me or isn't as lean as me does not mean she's making excuses. Maybe her real life is different, maybe her body ideals are not the same as mine, and that is okay. The world would be a very sad place if we all looked the same or, more importantly, if we were all judged on how many lunges we accomplished that day.

So how do we stop social media from skewing our thoughts and lives? How do we stop social media from making us too dang body negative? How can we learn to open up the old Instagram and feel inspired, without allowing it to make us feel less-than?

**Realize your body is just a vessel transporting your soul, heart, and brain.** Remember: the exterior is just *that*. It is just a bunch of flesh, and doesn't define who we are inside.

**Follow women who have different looks, different shapes, and different body types.** Seeing that not everyone is a social media model is very uplifting. Follow women who incorporate varying degrees of fitness and wellness in their lives and show that everyone has different experiences and stories. The more variety of greatness in the world, the merrier.

**Shift from self-criticism to inspiration.** If someone pops up on your feed who *you think* has a skinnier, leaner, more toned, more chiseled body than you, remember that is their journey, applaud them, comment on their post to help lift them up, and use them as inspiration, not comparison. Often, people flaunting such images have the lowest self-esteem and may be looking for validation. We tend to use those pics as fuel to beat ourselves up, but we can instead choose to lift them up, rather that internalizing their message.

**Make a list of things you are grateful for. Gratitude beats comparison.** If you find yourself engaging in negative self-talk with yourself, shift to something you're grateful for and write it down. Refer back to this list whenever you need to be reminded of what you love in life. *The comparison game is a slippery slope.*

**Realize that social media is the highlight reel, not the behind-the-scenes.** You see people's edited, filtered, photoshopped or best pics, not the pics of them after they ate a large pizza.

**Follow people who don't just post about fitness and their body.** If you like dogs (which I do!), follow accounts that post cute puppy pics, or anything that will make you smile and feel uplifted and inspired. If you like dancing, follow accounts that showcase various dance styles. Or if you like rock climbing, follow people who are traveling, going on different climbing expeditions, and partaking in adventures daily.

**Be proactive instead of reactive.** When you start comparing yourself to others in a negative way, you are only reacting to the situation. Instead of feeling down about your body, shut the internet off and go do something you enjoy. Set some goals for yourself and go crush them. Focus on you!

**Block, unfollow, delete, or just say "See ya" to those who are always bringing up these negative feelings or emotions about yourself and your body.** You don't need that in your life, and you can definitely control what you look at on the internet. If it truly isn't serving you — time to cut ties. Social media should be a positive and uplifting experience. Use it to HELP you in your fitness journey, not hinder you.

By controlling how social media affects our body image and ideals, we can stop the madness of trying to change and instead highlight, accept, and rock the shit out of our bodies!

Now I have to go take a butt selfie — it's been more than an hour and my Instagram followers will be wondering where I am! #justkidding

*I love my body. I am very much OK with it. I don't think artists are ever the ones who have a problem with it, it is other people.*

~ KELLY CLARKSON

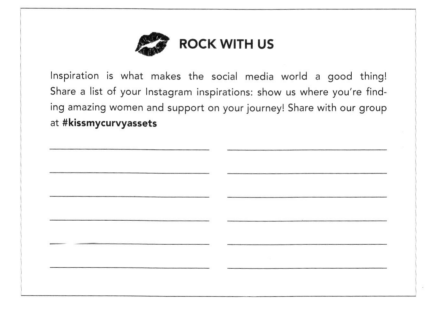

**ROCK WITH US**

Inspiration is what makes the social media world a good thing! Share a list of your Instagram inspirations: show us where you're finding amazing women and support on your journey! Share with our group at **#kissmycurvyassets**

## NOTES

_____
_____
_____
_____
_____
_____
_____
_____
_____
_____
_____
_____
_____
_____
_____
_____
_____
_____
_____
_____
_____
_____
_____
_____

# CHAPTER 4

# IT'S WHAT'S INSIDE THAT COUNTS - MASTER YOUR MINDSET

*I realize everybody wants what they don't have. But at the end of the day, what you have inside is much more beautiful than what's on the outside!*

~ SELENA GOMEZ

Every nutrition or fitness plan has its pros and cons, but for any plan to really work, you've got to get your mindset right. Shifting your mindset is the biggest factor in achieving your fitness goals and rockin' the shit out of your body! Most people start new fitness or nutrition programs with the worst state of mind possible: wanting to "fix" themselves. They jump into diets and exercise plans out of self-deprecation, all the while focusing on their "trouble" spots, calling themselves "fat," and feeling altogether less than. Obsessed with results, they focus on quick fixes and lose sight of sustainability.

What if we looked a little deeper, beyond just the tight booties and ripped abs? What if we dug a little deeper and focused within, internally . . . in the mind? What if our brain and emotions were so solid that our exterior fitness goals just happened organically, without forcing or extremes? We often work so hard on the surface that we forget to dive through the layers of skin and train the mindset.

What is mindset? Mindset is defined as: 1) an attitude, disposition, or mood and 2) an intention or inclination.[11]

But how does having a solid mindset really help us find our ideal bodies and reach our fitness goals? Let's first explore two different mindsets: a fixed mindset versus a growth mindset. The basic premise, introduced by Stanford University psychologist Carol Dweck, is that a fixed mindset is just that — fixed. In this mindset, creativity, character, intelligence, and performance are static. On the other hand, a growth mindset considers all of these characteristics to be flexible. Having a growth mindset is believing and knowing that habits can be worked on, trained, cultivated. Someone with a growth mindset will perceive failure as a tool that propels them toward growth, rather than as a setback.

When you understand this, you will come to realize that a person with a fixed mindset is predominantly focused on the external stuff. How they look, their bodies, the end result. An individual with a growth mindset, on the other hand, is focused on progress, not perfection. They give themselves the grace to celebrate their daily progress — small changes that develop into a long-term commitment over time.

# IT'S WHAT'S INSIDE THAT COUNTS...

Wouldn't it be so easy to just adopt the growth mindset and move ahead in our lives whenever we are faced with any challenges? Sadly, we become preprogrammed with a set of beliefs from our past experiences, some of which can even stem from our childhood. The beliefs we internalize from our childhood and life experiences are often irrational but can have a strong subconscious hold over us, significantly influencing and impacting our actions and decisions. For example, you commit to eating healthier — meal preps are done, clean grocery shopping lists are made and completed, there is even a solid meal plan in place, with all the recipes you could possibly crave and prepare with ease. You are making some solid changes to your overall nutrition, the ball is rolling, and you are excited and motivated to keep at it. But based on your past failures with healthy eating, deep down you believe that this time won't be any different. You bring the word "failure" with you. Cue the self-sabotage — you remember all the times you didn't succeed with healthy eating, fell off the wagon, and didn't follow through. Or you start thinking of excuses and reasons why this won't work again.

Sound familiar? Can we teach an old dog new tricks? Can we reprogram our minds? I have to let you in on a secret: YES. It is possible to break the shackles of a fixed mindset and to shift to a growth mindset.

Our thoughts and beliefs are powerful, as they cultivate our day-to-day reality. But guess what? We have the power to choose our beliefs. Just like we train our muscles to get stronger and gain lean muscle over time, we need to train our mind to create this shift. So once we change our mindset and reprogram our beliefs, what does this mean for our fitness goals and rockin' our body?

First things first — we have to change the way we think about ourselves and the way we talk to ourselves. Thoughts become words, which then become actions, which then become your reality. You get my drift? Saying things like "I can't" or "I failed" are not helping you to forge ahead with a new mindset. If we can work on reframing how we perceive failure and setbacks, we can create positive progress for ourselves.

For example, instead of viewing dieting setbacks as a completely failed mission, we can reframe that perspective to: _____ is what worked for me from that particular meal plan or diet, and _____ is what didn't work for me because _____. Now I can use what worked for me from this plan and combine it with something new. This is growth mindset in thought and sustained action. Accepting failure as part of our long-term progress and as a tool to help us grow is a key part of adopting a growth mindset and leaning into all the curveballs life throws at us. We are all bound to make mistakes or have some slip-ups with our nutrition or fitness goals (you are freakin human, y'know!), but it's how we deal with them that counts.

What do you do when you slip up? Are you the fixed mindset that blames, shames, and dwells? Or are you able to harness the power of your mind to stretch and grow beyond your comfort zone by speaking to yourself with kindness, optimism, and grace, saying, "Minor mistakes happen, I'm human, dust off and keep going." This reprogramming takes time and consistency. It's easy to want to slip back into the old negative fixed mindset.

Of course, it's easy to just say, "Change your way of thinking," or "Focus on mindset," but what are some actual strategies you can start to implement to get you REPROGRAMMING THE MIND? How do we ensure we don't slip back into old habits or keep falling back down the old rabbit hole of limiting beliefs? How can we change our mindset and be healthier, happier, and way more effective in terms of rocking the shit out of our bodies, for the long term?

**Change your goals.** Losing weight might be a result, but it shouldn't be the goal. Rather, your goals should be small and sustainable things over which you have full control — eating more veggies, drinking more water, or getting eight hours of sleep. These will yield a high success rate.

**Surround yourself with positivity.** Have people around you who support your goals and are uplifting for your spirit. This provides you an encouraging, emotionally healthy environment. Ask friends for support or help, and don't be afraid to enlist the help of a wellness coach.

**Food is not a reward or a punishment. It is a source of nourishment.** Making healthy choices is a way of practicing self-care. Food isn't a reward, and following your plan for a week doesn't mean you should have a binge-eating weekend to celebrate. Similarly, when you overdo it, you shouldn't use over-exercising or starving as a form of punishment. Nutrition and exercise are supposed to be good for your body. They should support you in looking and, more importantly, feeling your best.

**Take a deep breath.** Taking a few minutes at the beginning of your workout, or even at the beginning of your day, to slow down and simply inhale and exhale can help you set your intentions, connect with your body, and lower your stress response. It really is just the simple act of breathing. When was the last time you actually sat and focused on your breath? Take a nice long walk and just breathe. Slow down your breathing and close your eyes to feel the rise and fall of your belly and chest. Any time you feel the need to self-sabotage or notice negative feelings resurfacing — stop, and take a deep breath.

**Patience is a virtue.** Patience is so important when you have long-term fitness and wellness goals. To see sustainable results, slow and steady wins the race. Set smaller short-term goals, and think about the long-term picture. Remember, "Rome wasn't built in a day."

**Identify your "bad thoughts."** Identify the thoughts that get you into that negative space of feeling badly, and work to stop and change them. One common example is when you look in the mirror. What is that little voice in your head telling you? Another example is what you resort to when you become stressed. Does stress trigger your mind to automatically want food? You can easily make these thoughts stop by saying out loud, "STOP!" This then allows you time to insert more positive affirmations or better self-talk.

**Throw out the weight scale.** Many of us have learned to associate negative feelings with the number we see on the scale. But the scale is a random number generator that does not give us the bigger picture or show our true results. The scale is not the proper way to measure changes to your body, so put it away, smash it, or just walk by it without needing it to justify your hard work.

**Treat yourself like you would treat your best friend.** We would never talk to our best friends the way our inner voice talks to us. We are so hard on ourselves and not very nice to ourselves at all! Would you ever treat your bestie this way? You deserve the same respect and compassion you extend to the people closest to you. Be your own best friend first.

**Abandon the "foods are good or bad" mentality.** Somewhere along the line, we've learned to feel either proud or guilty about every food choice we make. But it's just food, and you shouldn't have to feel guilty about wanting the occasional cookie. Give yourself permission to have a glass of wine or a piece of chocolate cake. Rid yourself of the "cheat meal" or "good foods versus bad foods" mentality.

**Focus on the attainable.** Don't jump with both feet into a pool that's twenty feet deep. Set smaller goals that are more attainable. For example, if you aren't currently working out, it's reaching to say that you will go to the gym for two hours a day, six days a week! Start slow and steady. For example, shoot for twice a week for a month. Then build from there. If you know you don't have time to prep your own food, then look into enlisting the help of a food prep company for even half of your meals. Start where you are and build from there.

# IT'S WHAT'S INSIDE THAT COUNTS...

What about this whole concept of "It's what's inside that counts"? What if we could also reframe *why* we eat nourishing foods and move our bodies with exercise? What if it wasn't because we wanted to achieve a certain body type or level of lean? Let's talk about external motivation versus internal motivation.

External motivation reminds me of those people on social media who post every meal, every workout, every body part, constantly. Those looking for motivation from others' posts and comments. A person who feels motivated by external sources will train with the end goal of looking a certain way; they want to look good, fit into an outfit, undo years of over-indulging in a few months or even weeks, and almost always see this process as something to endure until a certain end point or stop date. They flock to the transformation challenges, overnight results, quick fixes. They're searching for one point when they'll achieve whatever it is they aspire to, like a goal weight. However, they're often unwilling to put in the effort and take the necessary steps to maintain that goal. They give up or move on to the next quick-fix or fad. We live in a world where this focus on external motivation is accepted, and often pushed on us. We are taught to set goals, and we all celebrate when we get there — no matter what it takes to get there. We love the before-and-after pictures, but we forget about what comes next.

Then there is internal motivation. This means that we have goals, but they don't have an end point. We develop new habits that are sustainable for life. We can be motivated by little achievements made daily, monthly, yearly, and over a lifetime. With this mindset, our goals are often just things we can continue improving on, year after year. Our focus is often just on trying to get better, to feel better on the inside, to live a longer, more enjoyable life. An internally motivated person doesn't worry about numbers on the scale or end dates; they have a bigger picture in mind. An internally motivated person nourishes themselves and trains from within, which then supports long-term health and wellness. They refuse to hurt their health for a number on the scale or short-term fitness goal.

What motivates you to exercise and eat healthier foods? If you reached your goals tomorrow, would you stop right away, or would you make more goals and be back the next day to keep seeing long-term changes? What if you could truly focus on what matters most? Ensuring your heart is beating at full capacity. Waking up and moving without pain and with ease. Adding years to your life to enjoy more time with your partner, children and grandchildren, and friends and to travel. Living every day with great digestion, a healthy sex life, and just being happy. What if doing all these things ensured that your external goals also fell into place naturally? It doesn't happen the other way around.

I often see women train externally, without the proper mindset and inner work. Their results are short-term, superficial, and usually not achieved in the healthiest ways. On the other hand, if you truly do shift your mindset to a growth mindset and find your internal motivation, getting the body you have always wanted will just be icing on your already delicious cake. (Mmmm, cake . . . wait, where was I?) Believe you have a rockin" body, and you will rock the shit out of that body. At the end of the day, this is the key to long-term fitness and health. After all, as the popular adage goes, *"It's what's on the inside that counts."*

*We all have imperfections. But I'm human and you know, it's important to concentrate on the qualities besides outer beauty.*

~ BEYONCE KNOWLES

## ROCK WITH US

Now that you've been given a list of tools to help get you in the right mindset, tell us what you're going to start focusing on to start **ROCKIN' THOSE CURVES AND ASSETS!!!** Send us pics and links at **#kissmycurvyassets**

_____

_____

_____

## NOTES

_____
_____
_____
_____
_____
_____
_____
_____
_____
_____
_____
_____
_____
_____

## NOTES

# CHAPTER 5

# DIVORCE THE SCALE

*Being a healthy woman isn't about getting on a scale or measuring your waistline. We need to start focusing on what matters - how we feel, and how we feel about ourselves.*

~ MICHELLE OBAMA

It's early morning, and you bounce out of bed full of positive energy to take on the day. You disrobe in the bathroom and stand naked in front of this square metal object. Filled with hope and optimism, you take a deep breath and close your eyes, and as you exhale every last ounce of air in your lungs, you step forward to stand on it. You tilt your head down in anticipation of what you are about to see. In an instant, that small glimmer of hope you felt is shattered as you open your eyes to that number staring back at you. One little number that holds every single ounce of your self-worth, self-esteem, and self-confidence in its hands. That very moment you decided to step on that square metal box, just like that, you have decided things about yourself.

For me, that little song and dance was a part of my life for thirty years. I remember the first time I stepped on it. I was a twelve-year-old swimmer and was at a local recreation centre and saw this glowing object in the corner of the change room. Little did I know that stepping on it just once would spark a toxic and abusive relationship that would span over three decades.

The modern scale was invented in the 1770s by a man named Richard Salter.[12] Thanks, Richard, for single-handedly ruining the self-esteem and body images of trillions of women everywhere. Little did he know that the invention of this little gadget would birth a whole slew of insanity for women all over the world. Why are we stepping on the scale to measure our own progress and quality of health and wellbeing? I mean, the scale can be encouraging on some days, yet so defeating on most other days.

We often associate the number that comes up on the scale to either "failing" or "succeeding," but it doesn't really tell us the whole story. Your bodyweight is not a reflection of who you are — your strength, intelligence, kindness, beauty, and worth. In fact, your weight alone does not give you the complete picture of your true health. True health comes in all shapes and sizes, so why do we strive for a number? How did we even come up with this number? Why do we attach our body image so closely to that one number? Too often, we believe what the scale is telling us, rather than what is in front of our own eyes, and we end up feeling so discouraged and frustrated rather than celebrating our successes.

For twenty-seven years, I have been coaching women in the fitness and wellness industry and have come to this conclusion: our relationship with the scale is a toxic one. It's a bad marriage! One person (you) is trying their best. You are putting in the effort and giving so much of yourself. You are trusting and letting the other person control your self-worth. Then there is the other person in the relationship (the scale), who thrives on preying on your weaknesses, bullying you into believing they hold all of the power and control over your well-being. They have the power to dictate how you will feel or act. That person (or scale) continues to degrade you and your sense of self, making you feel you are less than enough, beating you down, and taking away your self-confidence or self-worth with one little number. Day after day, week after week, month after month, year after year.

Just like with any toxic relationship or marriage that strips you down little by little, it's time to cut ties and divorce the scale!

Before we break up with the scale, let's talk about why it's so toxic to our well-being. It's simple, really. This random number generator:

**Has the power to set our mood for the day**. It causes us such mental and physical stress when we don't see the number we long for or anticipated.

**Strips down our self-worth.** We base whether we are good enough or not on one number!

**Hinders our ability to listen to our body.** How often have you experienced this? You're feeling so good, happy, exercising hard, nourishing your body with amazing foods, and noticing your stomach feels flatter - only to weigh yourself and wham! In an instant, that small feeling of success is crushed!

**Creates an unhealthy obsession with food and can lead to disordered eating patterns.** We get on that terrible metal object and when it spits out a number that doesn't show losses, we punish ourselves by taking away more food or adding extreme exercise in order to lower it. We begin associating that number not moving with needing less food or with food being bad.

**Doesn't give us the bigger picture of true health.** The scale doesn't take into account the whole story of what our body is telling us in terms of biofeedback (which is just a fancy word for all the signs our body gives us, like energy, sleep, clarity, mood, digestion, skin, sex drive, and our general feelings).

The scale doesn't take into account the bigger picture of our true health and fitness results. It can't measure the following:

**Our sodium levels.** For example, eating a saltier meal the night before would yield an increased weight on the scale the next morning. This isn't an increase in your body fat levels, but rather water retention or temporary swelling.

**Our menstrual cycles and hormone levels.** Some women bloat excessively or gain water weight heading into their periods, and this can cause the numbers on the scale to increase. Again, it doesn't mean a change in body fat, and it's temporary.

**Our stress levels and adrenal health.** During times of stress, whether prolonged or isolated, our body can get inflamed and retain water. This causes that little number to increase and trick us into thinking we are failing.

**Our quality of sleep.** Lack of sleep or restless nights can also cause our bodies to retain excess water, which results in an inaccurate reading on that mean scale!

**Climate changes and daily temperature.** The temperature in warm climates is another factor that can add to water retention and short-term swelling.

**Hydration or dehydration.** Our body is mainly water, so a change in hydration can cause significant weight fluctuations that have nothing to do with body fat gain or losses.

**Changes in body composition.** This is a big one! When our body composition changes due to various circumstances, those changes are not accurately measured by a scale. For instance, when we strength train, we gain lean muscle, which is more dense than fat tissue, hence increasing the numbers on the scale. Since lean muscle takes up less space than body fat and is more metabolically active (which is fancy wording for burning more calories at a more rapid rate), we should actually aspire to the increasing numbers on the scale when we are trying to add more lean muscle. I often use the story of the Jell-o and the rock. Everyone knows what a big blob of Jell-o looks like. It's all flowy, and jiggly, and light. Then you have a rock, which is small, but dense, heavy, and hard. Put the rock on the scale and it weighs much more than the jello, but which would you want to be? I would take the heavy rock any day! Does the number on the scale really make a difference? While many of us focus on the pounds we are losing, what's important is how much fat we're losing, which is something the scale can't tell us.

Why do we continue to let a hunk of metal determine our mood, self-worth, progress, self-confidence, and state of mind? It's time to serve the paperwork - it's time for a divorce! Changing our lifestyle habits are hard enough without the added pressure of losing a certain number of pounds each week.

So when will we finally say goodbye to this relationship that is beating us down? What other methods can we use to truly gauge our progress? How can we replace that dreaded routine of weighing ourselves and waiting for the metal bully to generate that number? Let's start by replacing the scale and use the following methods to stay attuned our true results:

**How do your clothes fit (and I don't mean the skinny jeans in the closet from 2001)?** If your pants are feeling looser or if zipping them up feels easier, it could be revealing inches lost, even if the scale may be lying and saying you haven't changed.

**Has your digestion improved?** By selecting a nutrition plan that nourishes our body, we can ensure that our digestion improves, our stomach loses that inflamed and bloated feeling, and of course, we feel much happier.

**How's your strength and endurance?** By focusing on how we feel during each workout, we can gauge whether our endurance levels, strength, and form have improved — all of which are indicators of true progress. The boost in self-confidence also helps!

**How is your energy?** Notice the difference in your energy levels. Are you feeling more at ease in your body and with yourself? Are you more agile, motivated, inspired, and overall in a more aware and confident state of mind? Seeing results means flowing through your daily activities with ease and with a sustained momentum of intentional energy — again, an indicator of our progression.

**Focus on behaviors, not numbers.** This will make incorporating and implementing a lifestyle change more natural, sustainable, and better for long-term progress and results. When you focus on the long-term benefits of a lifestyle overhaul, such as exercising regularly (whatever regularly means for you — every day or a few times a week) or choosing foods that fuel your body properly, not only will you yield results but you will also increase the quality of your life. You reduce the risk of disease, lengthen your lifespan, and improve your overall health.

**Bare it all and own it all.** There's nothing like a photograph to see how your body is really responding, so take pictures instead of the dreaded weigh-ins. A picture is worth a thousand words, and with some high tech apps out there now, you can actually create side-by-side pictures to measure your progress during your health and fitness journey. The numbers on the scale may be telling you a story in which nothing has changed, but when you take the side-by-side photos, you may see a more defined and shaped waistline, toned legs, and just an overall leaner physique. If you don't want pictures, use the "Naked Test." Stand naked in front of your mirror and truly look at how your body is transforming (but don't let the little negative-Nelly in your head be too hard on yourself, or you will miss the subtle changes that have been taking place week to week).

**Let go of the body composition ideals laid out by society and instead create your own.** Often society's numbers are unrealistic, require insane restrictions to obtain, and just throw us into a negative self-image spiral. You do you — create how you want to look. You don't need to play into the insane number games that society pushes onto us.

I'm talking to you as my best friend now. If I saw my best friend in an abusive relationship, I would save her. I would demand she break up with the abuse, ask for more in life, see her self-worth as important. I would scream at her, shake her, and tell her to get a divorce. So I'm telling you, as my best friend — let go of that number so that you can find long-term success and the body you have always wanted.

Let's regain control of how we look and feel about our bodies without the use of this small metal piece of junk. It won't be easy; it will take consistent change and a conscious effort.

Picture your morning tomorrow — you get out of bed, feeling positive and ready to take on the day. You enter the bathroom, disrobe like any other day. This time, empower yourself to look down at the empty space where that metal object, the scale, once was. Now you are beginning a new chapter, reaching toward *your* fitness goals on *your* terms, and taking back the power and control the scale once held over your well-being. You are beginning this new day reaching for *your* fitness goals or body ideals with more positivity, less stress, and a zest to take on the day. You zip up those size __ jeans with ease, nourish your body with an amazing breakfast, and thank yourself for finally getting that divorce! You consciously uncoupled (haha!) from the once-glorious scale. There's no anger or resentment over the years or decades of self-love that the scale may have robbed from you. You had a long run together, but now you have decided you need more and deserve better. Breathe in the amazing energy and feel the weight lifted off you by ending that rollercoaster relationship. Thank yourself for divorcing that piece of metal. You are free — free to finally focus on your health and wellness without the burden of numbers. It's all about quality instead of quantity, and you, my friend, will soon see an endless amount of true progress! Who is ready to rock the shit out of their body with me, free from this numbers-game mind screw?!

*My weight? It is what it is. You could get hit by a bus tomorrow. It's about being content, and sometimes other priorities win.*

~ MELISSA MCCARTHY

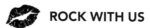 **ROCK WITH US**

Show us the image of you throwing your scale in the garbage, smashing it with a sledge hammer, waving buh-bye as it sails through the air and into the trash. Then (you know it) **SEND US THE PIC** at **#kissmycurvyassets!**

## NOTES

_____

_____

_____

_____

_____

_____

_____

_____

_____

_____

_____

_____

_____

_____

_____

_____

_____

_____

_____

## NOTES

# CHAPTER 6

# BREAK UP
# WITH FAD DIETS

*If anybody even tries to whisper the word*
*"diet," I'm like "You can go fuck yourself!"*

~ JENNIFER LAWRENCE

### *Dear Diet, It's not me, it's you. I just don't think it's going to work between us. You're boring, tasteless, and I just can't stop cheating on you.*

Hands up, nod your head, no judgements here . . . Have you tried a fad diet before? How did it go? How did you feel? Are you still doing the same diet now? Did you keep off the promised weight? Did anyone get injured or killed while you were on it? #couldhappen

If you are like me, you have been so excited and optimistic about the empty promises given by these diets, and then sadly your world got crushed when you not only couldn't maintain the losses but often were worse off than when you started. (I actually get hungry just thinking about being on a fad diet — stomach growling and yelling, "NOOOOO!") There is a huge secret that the weight loss industry doesn't want you to know, so first they feed you things like:

- Special diet protocols

- Blood-type programming

- Cutting out certain foods or macronutrients. (fancy terminology for type of food - protein, carbs or fats)

- Secret pills, juices, cleanses, and supplements (usually costly $$$)

- Multi-level marketing businesses

- Transformation challenges promising overnight results

I'm going to let you in on the secret . . . It's all a BUNCH OF BULLSHIT! There is no special trick or product that guarantees long-term, sustainable fitness and nutrition. However, the weight loss industry wants you to believe there is so you keep paying big $$$! The more you keep believing, the more money they make!

Enter the fad diet. A fad diet or "diet cult" is a diet that makes promises of weight loss or other health advantages, such as longer life, without backing by solid science; in many cases, these diets are characterized by highly restrictive or unusual food choices.[13] A fad diet is an eating plan that becomes popular quickly. Fad diets often promise dramatic, unrealistic weight loss results.

Many are designed to take advantage of people's willingness to "try anything" to lose weight, look and feel better, and reduce their risk for diseases and other health problems.

Many fad diets become popular because they do produce short-term weight loss quickly. Our society tends to have the "I want it, and I want it now mentality!" However, most of these diets do not result in long-term weight loss success. They often are unhealthy — in fact, some fad diets can severely jeopardize your health by promoting unhealthy eating habits that don't meet nutritional recommendations.[14] They may provide far fewer daily calories than normal (think "crash" diets), resulting in weight loss that stems mainly from a loss of water weight and lean muscle mass, not body fat.

It's difficult for most people to maintain any diet that drastically restricts their food choices or requires them to eat unusual foods, very little food, or the same foods day after day. Therefore, people who lose weight on a fad diet usually gain the weight back — and then some. Even worse, the damage done to their internal systems, such as their metabolic rate, is sometimes irreversible. Most of these diets cannot be considered long-term solutions for sustained weight loss. They just provide a quick fix, a band-aid solution.

Let's talk about the history of the "Fad Diet," since it clearly isn't something new. I am not going to list them all (it would take up way more than a chapter of this book!), but I will tell you some of the ones that stand out to me throughout history.[15]

**1820**: The Water and Vinegar Diet (which I believe has recently made a comeback in the form of apple cider vinegar).

**1925**: Lucky Strike Cigarettes "Reach for a lucky, instead of a sweet," campaign, actually promoting smoking as an appetite suppressant. WTF were people thinking!

**1930s**: The Grapefruit Diet — This is still around almost 100 years later.

**1950s:** Cabbage Soup Diet — I actually tried and failed at this one — and had BAD GAS and severe bloating!

**1970**: The Sleeping Beauty Diet (no, this wasn't invented by us tired moms) — invites medical sedation (that's right, being put under!) and is rumored to have been tried by Elvis (I can't make this shit up!).

**1975**: The Cookie Diet — A Florida doctor invented a cookie with amino acids (how in the heck did I miss this one?!).

**1975**: The Last Chance Diet — A liquid of predigested animal byproducts ("meat smoothie") later pulled off the market when people died . . . (seriously, who falls for this bullshit?!).

**1977**: Slimfast — A shake for breakfast, a shake for lunch, and a sensible dinner (I did it, and the shakes were disgusting and I actually vomited from them!).

**1979**: Dexatrim — A diet drug that hit the shelves in drug stores and was later pulled after being linked to strokes (thank goodness I didn't try this one!).

**1985**: The Caveman Diet (don't worry, this makes a comeback in 2010 as what we know as The Paleo Diet).

**1988**: Wearing a pair of size ten jeans and pulling a bucket of fat in a wagon, Oprah loses sixty-seven pounds on the liquid diet.

**1992**: Jeff Atkins launches the Atkins Diet, touting low carb, high protein foods like bacon and butter (the inventor later died of heart disease, clearly someone I don't want to take dieting advice from!).

**2000**: The Macrobiotic Diet — aka the "complicated seaweed and food-combining diet that makes you buy a whole new stove and cook all your foods only to a certain temp" diet (Madonna and Gwyneth Paltrow made this one famous).

**2006**: The Master Cleanse — Beyonce promoted this one, which involved drinking hot water, lemon juice, maple syrup, and cayenne for ten days. (I did this for three days and actually passed out at work, out cold!).

**2011**: The Human Chorionic Gonadotropin (HCG) Diet — This involved a strict 500-calorie-a-day regimen while taking drops or injections of a fertility drug (it promises a weight loss of twenty-one pounds in twenty-one days . . . the fine print should read "and then gain back thirty pounds!").

I honestly could go on and on. The Baby Food Diet, the "Eat Right For Your Blood Type" diet, all the various protein shakes, meal replacement shakes, and weight loss pills and supplements... It's endless.

Fad diets or extremes don't work in the long term because they limit the quantity and the variety of food you can eat. While in this state of caloric deprivation, restriction, and insanity, women become depleted, tired, hungry, and angry. In addition, women can also experience hormonal imbalances, adrenal fatigue, and suffer from emotional disturbances, low libido, or loss of libido altogether. Sounds fun! Definitely a recipe for disaster.

With deprivation or extreme diets, we often make food an object of reward, attention, or emotional value. We then behave much like a toddler who seeks comfort from her "blankie" or "soother" for emotional relief. Turning to food for emotional comfort then becomes something we view as a form of positive reinforcement. It ends up being less about the actual taste or value of the food, and more about the desired emotional reward. We become obsessed with thoughts such as *When I am done this diet, I cannot wait to go to that new all-you-can-eat sushi restaurant*, or *Few more days till we head off to Mexico on vacation, it'll be worth it, I can eat to my heart's content. After all, that is why I'm doing this cleanse or diet, so that I can eat whatever I want while vacationing.*

This new obsession and emotional awareness leads to an intense focus on food as reward, followed by further mental and emotional torment.

Diets, when unsustainable, often leave you feeling frustrated, or have you spinning your wheels, and make you think you are a failure. Repeat after me: "I didn't fail these programs — they failed me!" Or be it better yet, "I didn't fail these diets, they were set up to make me fail!" These fads, extremes, and packaged insanity are part of that thirty-three billion dollar industry that just wants to kick you when you are down. If you found *your* balance in your health and wellness, and actually started loving your body, you wouldn't need the next great fad or trend to make you feel whole or enough, and big businesses would stop profiting from our pain. It's like we are all drowning in water, unable to swim, and they throw us a rope, which in this case is the fad diet. However, the rope is actually not whole or firm — it has little cuts in it and fibers are coming loose. Of course, sooner or later it will break, and then WHAM! We are treading water, still unable to be saved, until the next life boat or rope (fad diet) pulls up and offers a brief but weak reprieve.

As women, we often jump into quick, extreme, intense, and various fad diets, without realizing that it's the small, daily shifts in our lifestyles that will lead to major long-term progress and results. So instead of taking on the "all-or-nothing" mentality, how do we spot these phonies in the dieting world?

**Most fad diets use the words "good" vs "bad."** This implies that you do something wrong when you consume the foods from the "bad" list. Eating a food should not make you feel bad. Ever.

**Most fad diets have an END DATE.** You only have to make it ___ amount of weeks — because it is impossible to maintain the diet forever, and then you blow up like a beluga whale when you go back to "normal ways of life and eating."

**Some fad diets require the purchase of extras** such as fancy pills, supplements, shakes, juices, etc. Stripping it down and just keeping it about real food, without the need for any of these extras, is the key to long-term fitness. There are some tasty protein shakes out there that make it easier to eat healthier options, but you shouldn't be required to purchase them to be healthy or lose weight.

**Some fad diets require the participants to sell products or get their friends to sign up (fad / multi-level marketing in disguise).** MLM (multi-level marketing companies) often prey on people who are trying to make money, while promoting products that may not be as they are promised. I won't put down all MLMs — there have been some great products out there — but when you have that dollar and sales attached to health, my back goes against the wall and I question the product's legitimacy. MLMs are usually about sales, and less about quality or sustainability. Thus why we see many MLM products come and then go just as quickly. They phase out because it truly was about the corporate profit and less about providing quality products for long-term fitness and health. In the end, you shouldn't focus on *products* to help you embrace your body and find long-term fitness. The twenty strategies I'm laying out in this book can do a lot more for you than any pill or shake. You're welcome for saving you all that money!

**Fad diets often have a label attached to them,** and a cult-like mentality.

**Fad diets often make you hangry (meaning hungry and angry), sick or mean.** Because they are extremes.

**Fad diets make exaggerated claims**. Lose ten pounds in ten days, or lose four dress sizes in a week.

Quick results mean short term-gains, which don't last and aren't sustainable. Below are some more staggering statistics about fad diets.[16]

- In 2010, fifty-four percent of adults said that they were currently on a diet. That's the highest number since survey results were first collected in 1986.

- US weight-loss market revenues totaled nearly sixty-one billion to date.

- Australian research has shown that young girls who diet at severe levels are 18 times more likely to develop an eating disorder within six months.

- Losing weight is consistently one of the top resolutions made at the start of every new year.

- Sixty-five percent of people who successfully complete a fad diet will end up gaining all of that weight back.

- More than ninety-five percent of people relapse from a diet in five years or less.

- The average American adult tries to implement a fad diet four times per year.

- Twenty-five percent of Americans will give up on their weight loss goals within two weeks.

Okay, so we need to steer clear of fad diets or trends, but what do we do if we still want to be healthy, lose weight, and reach our fitness goals? Here are some tips that will serve as a guide so that you know you are on the right track to find *your* healthy balance and blueprint:

**If it tastes good, makes you feel good, and supports your goals - EAT IT!** Learn to fuel your body from within and act from a place of love and not deprivation.

**Whole foods are always ideal for digestion, but they are not the be-all-end-all.** Try to nourish yourself from the inside, and your outside fitness goals will follow. Have you ever eaten something that just made your stomach hurt? It's not fun to eat something that causes issues with your tummy. Paying attention to your body's cues after you have consumed certain foods makes it easy to know what actually makes you feel good.

**Avoid words like "can't" or "rules" and replace them with words like "choose" and "variety."** Don't let anyone or any plan tell you what you can or can't do.

Learn to reframe and repair your relationship with food by breaking up with extreme fad diets and becoming conscious and intentional of how you nourish and refuel your body. This will help you find the long-term success and healthy body image you desire, and learn to rock the shit out of your body!

*I'm not going to starve just to be thin. I want to enjoy life, and I can't if I'm not eating and miserable.*

~ KATE UPTON

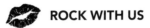 

### ROCK WITH US

List all of the fad diets you have tried in the past on a piece of paper – take a screenshot of them. Hashtag us at **#kissmycurvyassets** to show you accepting that you tried, but are now willing to have that list be your last list for fads! Tear it up, throw it out, turn it into a paper airplane and let it fly into the world and away from you. Help us say so long to the toxic food cycle!

## NOTES

# CHAPTER 7

# STOP GIVING A SHIT ABOUT OTHER PEOPLE'S OPINIONS — JUST DO YOU!

*To all of you that have something nasty to say about me, or other women that are built like me . . . I have one thing to say to you. Kiss my fat ass!*

~ TYRA BANKS

*That hot pink outfit with the red lace trim — I want to wear it, but what will people think of me? That skirt I just purchased fits quite snug, will people think I look chunky in it? I'm so nervous, I have to get up and speak in front of that group, will they notice I've gained ten pounds? Oh, I know they will be talking and laughing about my weight gain all night. Those whispers and laughter, the finger pointing - I bet you anything they must be talking about me.*

Does this inner dialogue sound familiar? This was me for most of my life. I worried constantly about others' opinions and I let them define me — what I wore, the color of my hair. My fear of weight gain was directly handcuffed to the opinions of others.

What kinds of fears or judgments hold you back or continue to hinder your progress? Why do the opinions of those around us, including perfect strangers, matter to us so much? Why do we live our lives and take action (or don't) based on how we expect those around us to react? By doing so, we give away our power to those around us and live from an unempowered stance. It can feel as though we are walking on a tightrope or even walking on eggshells, gingerly, delicately, without any direction, for fear of ridicule, judgment, and the all-consuming opinion of the "community." We don't always take action on what lights us up because we are too afraid. Too afraid to make a misstep in the wrong direction — *Oh, but what if I lose my footing? What will others think of me?*

When was the last time you did something for yourself without considering the opinions of others? I have to be truly honest — this chapter is very emotional for me, not only because I experienced such emotional beatdowns, I also allowed others to hold my self-worth in the palm of their hand. It is also emotional because I continue to coach and guide women on how to break free from this prison of letting others control their sense of self-worth. Social media adds a whole new dimension, allowing people worldwide to have a say in how we act, and to spew hate and venom in our direction for no reason and with no repercussions. Based off my personal experiences, I want to assure you that the moment you truly let go and stop caring about what others think of you, when you own your power and stop giving a shit about others' opinions — that is when you will find your long-term fitness goals with flow and ease, and can begin to truly rock your body!

Here are some easy strategies to not give a shit what others think:

**The negative comments someone makes are on them and say more about them than about you. Sweetheart, it's not you, it's them.** The internet is famous for random strangers posting cruel and false comments (some random stranger even called me a "man" the other day on my Instagram!). Criticism about the way we look, what we eat or don't eat, what we wear or don't wear — constant body shaming. Cruelty at its finest. These things say more about the person posting the comment than they do about you. I remember when my two-year-old daughter was at our local playground and some older kids yelled at her, pushed her down, and said, "We don't want to play with you, you are ugly and stupid!" Instead of smacking them (which did come to mind, but would have been wrong of me, and I didn't want the jail time), I scooped her up and told her, "Don't worry, honey. Those kids don't have parents who love them." I meant it. For someone, even children, to be that cruel and upsetting to a little child says much more about them and their issues than about anything my daughter had done. It's terribly sad that some people have nothing better to do with their time than try to tear others down.

**Be true to yourself. Never sell yourself to the devil. You do you.** Some people will see your passion, your truth, and in this you will find true connections. Once I finally stopped caring so much about everyone's opinions and followed my heart, my life got significantly better. Never underestimate the beautiful power and freedom that washes over you when you commit to being true to yourself. By doing so, you will be surrounded by those who not only accept you but love you for who you are.

**This is your one life. I repeat, you only get one life. There are no re-dos.** During my college years, I had a placement at a seniors' centre, volunteering and getting to know people in their eighties and nineties. The women would say to me, "Oh Lori, just eat the damn cake, life is too short." They wanted me to stop carrying around my tupperware container of boiled chicken and broccoli, worrying about being a size four, and live a little instead! These older and wiser women would tell me stories of how they dieted their lives away and now as they neared the last days of their lives, their one piece of advice to young twenty-somethings like me at the time was . . . just eat the damn cake! When you can put things into perspective and realize that we only get one life, it makes it easier to stop caring so much about what other people think and to be true to yourself.

**Think — really think — about the absolute worst-case scenario. What's holding you back from doing the things you want to do?** I always wanted to write, to share my twenty-seven years of experience in this crazy fitness industry, but I was worried my book would flop. I was worried about being judged. Then I had a revelation. If I write from the heart, be true to what I know, and just put myself out there, the worst-case scenario is that I will reach some people and others will dislike me or the book. Meh. I know that my message and book will reach the people it is meant to guide and help. Heck, if this book hits a chord and helps just one person, then it is a true success to me. What is the worst thing that will happen if you do (insert whatever it is you want to do)? Remember the movie *The Hangover*, when Mr. Chow says, "But did you die!?" Will your worst-case scenario inflict pain or death? Chances are no, it won't! Some people will always be ignorant assholes, so the solution is so simple: Fuck em! (yep, I'm that passionate about this subject that I'm pulling out the F Bomb!) The next time you're hesitant to do something or take a risk because you're afraid of what other people will think, stop and ask yourself, "What's the worst-case scenario if I do this?" Chances are it's not that bad. And I can almost guarantee that you'll be worse off if you do or don't do things because you're more concerned with what others will think.

**Remove sources of negativity, ASAP!** Remember the unfollow, delete, and block social media chapter? That is to help you purge your life of negative, toxic people. If someone is bringing you down — sever ties! If someone is starting drama — avoid them! Separate yourself from the crazies and those who don't let you be yourself! If someone makes hurtful or rude comments about something you post on the internet, delete it or don't acknowledge it. (that little button that says "BLOCK" is my best friend) No good can come from feeding into the madness and negativity. I have always said, "You can't reason with crazy!"

**Trust the opinions of close, true friends, and ignore the rest. And more than anything, trust yourself.** Have a few select people whom you trust. The ones you know will tell you in the changeroom at the mall that those jeans make you look fatter than you are. The ones who aren't afraid to let loose, without hurting your feelings. Have a few close people you can confide in, people who you know have your best interest at heart. My best friend Patti is one who I know will always tell me if I am out of line, or wearing an outfit that doesn't show off my complete hotness to its fullest. Once she was going to do something really stupid and I threatened to go over to her house and smack her out of the insanity.

She has my back, and I have hers. And most of all, I have my own back — I am not afraid to trust my own instincts. Total strangers don't get to have that power over me anymore!

**Some people are going to dislike you, and there's nothing you can do about it.** Don't waste your time trying to get everyone to like you, because it's impossible. This is one I am carrying with me through this book — I will have some likes, and some people can take me or leave me, and that is okay. The world is a big place, and if I can empower even just one person with my message, then this book did its job. Let's all spend our time and energy living a powerful and happy life, using our abilities, gifts, and talents to make the world and people around us feel better.

Okay, so now we don't give a shit what others think anymore. But will not giving a shit alone truly help us achieve our own body ideals or our long-term fitness goals? Will giving less fucks about what people think of us truly help us move forward to embrace, accept, and rock the shit out of our bodies? Well, just like anything else in life you want to master, it will require consistent action and effort. Here are some amazing things that will happen When we master how to stop giving a shit about what other people think:

**We have no fears.** We can feel good about ourselves and, for the first time, take control of our own body ideals and look however we want to look without fear of judgment. We can block out others' opinions and can listen to our gut instinct more.

**We learn to say no.** We can avoid the fads and extremes when we know they don't feel right or even healthy to us. We can stop pretending to like something just because we are afraid to disappoint someone. And we can stop forcing ourselves to conform to mass society.

**We smell bullshit from a mile away.** We can sense when we are being lied to or manipulated, or when someone is trying to control us or influence our decision.

**We stop needing excuses.** When someone tries to sell us on the next fad or extreme, or tell us we need to try to fit a certain mold, we just say no. Thanks, but no thanks.

**We forget the word "fail."** When we stop caring about what others think, we take momentous leaps in our journey and gain more courage and boldness with each choice we make. We aren't afraid to mess up, and we don't listen to the harsh criticism of others. We listen more to that little voice in our own heart and block out the noise that is everyone else.

**We stop letting toxic people into our lives and only surround ourselves with good people.** We have no more time for toxic people and drama. We can be pickier about who gets our precious time and energy.

**We find more happiness.** We get to define what happiness means to us and can put happiness at the top of our priority list.

**We can stop worrying so much and focus on our own goals and what we truly desire.** We can stop worrying about the little imperfections and insecurities that once haunted us. We are no longer in competition with anyone but ourselves.

**Our confidence soars!** When we don't worry about living up to society's standards, we can be more confident. We move with a self-assured and empowered stance in the direction of our own goals!

Is it really that simple? Is it truly possible to let go of all the baseless opinions and stop caring about what others think and find our body ideals and goals? YES! Try it and see what happens! It is so liberating to just stop giving a shit.

As I end this chapter, I want to share a story. My twelve-year-old son is a big time dancer. Hip hop, lyrical, contemporary, ballet, jazz, musical theatre. He does it all, regardless of what anyone thinks of him. At school, when the kids tease him for dancing instead of playing hockey or soccer, he just shrugs his shoulders. He knows he loves dancing, and if "boys aren't supposed to do it," then he asks, "Why not?" His favorite color is purple, even when the rest of the boys tease him and tell him it should be blue instead. He loves wearing the color pink, even when the other boys tell him it's a "girl" color.

I love this attitude, and as his mom, I can take credit for instilling in him the belief that he can do whatever he wants to do, that it doesn't matter what anyone else thinks, that you do you! I also love to show him when we are out in public that I, too, do not care what anyone thinks of me. There is the saying: *"Dance like no one's watching."* I realized I actually don't like this saying. So, I have changed it, and my son agrees with me. Let's dance like everyone's watching, and not give a shit what they think!

So, when we are in public, we dance. We break out in a full hip hop dance routine in Walmart when we hear a good song come over the sound system. We do ballet twirls in the grocery store (which often makes people smile). We sing at the top of our lungs when we hear a song we like, without worrying if we are pitch perfect, not giving a shit about who's watching — I mean, this isn't *American Idol*. This embarrasses my teenage daughter, since she doesn't understand the need to do a full jazz routine at the zoo or the movies. But we love just being us. It makes us happy, living our lives without fear of judgements.

How liberating would this be to implement in your life, with your body, your body ideals, and how you feel every day? It would eliminate the mental and emotional load that so many of us have carried with us for too long, and enable us to find the long-term success we desire while rocking the shit out of our bodies. So the next time you are out, try busting a move in the line of the grocery store — dance like everyone's watching, and don't give a shit about what they think.

> *I've been through my highs, I've been through my lows; I've been through the gamut of all things in this business. Being too thin, Being bigger. I've been criticized for being on both sides of the scale. It's noise I block out automatically. I love my body.*

~ CHRISTINA AGUILERA

---

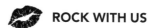 **ROCK WITH US**

Video yourself doing something silly like dancing at the grocery store or bank teller line up! Hashtag **#kissmycurvyasssets** and let's show the community how you are doing you, Boo!

---

## NOTES

_____

_____

_____

## NOTES

---

---

---

---

---

---

---

---

---

---

---

---

---

---

---

---

---

---

---

---

---

---

---

---

---

---

---

---

---

---

# CHAPTER 8

# FIND YOUR FOUR S'S - SELF-ACCEPTANCE, SELF-LOVE, SELF-ESTEEM, AND SELF-CARE

*If your self-esteem really does depend on how you look you're always going to be insecure. There's no way you can get around it because you are going to age. Even if you get that perfect body you're going to get older and older and older. You can't avoid it. So you have to somehow, at some point, take control and shift the focus and decide who you are, what you can contribute to the world, what you do and say, is so much more important than how you look.*

~ PORTIA DE ROSSI

We are not our bodies. Our bodies are the vessels that transports our souls around. How would it feel to find immense acceptance, love, esteem, and worth, so we can control how our exterior was seen? What if we were not defined by the size of our butts, the flatness of our tummies, or the width of our thighs? What if that was just the surface and who we truly are — our essence, our beauty — is more than skin deep?

Sounds easy, right? Love yourself on the inside and the external goals will organically follow. But how do we even do that? How do we stop our bodies from defining us and instead allow them to just be our vessels? To do that, we need to find our four S's: self-acceptance, self-love, self-esteem, and self-care.

## SELF-ACCEPTANCE

Self-acceptance is 1) the act or state of accepting oneself or 2) the act or state of understanding and recognizing one's own abilities and limitations.[17] In short, self-acceptance is your satisfaction or happiness with yourself. It plays a crucial part in how we perceive ourselves. People who have self-acceptance usually have a positive attitude, accept their strengths as well as areas that need improvement, are not critical or confused about their identity, and don't wish they were different than who they are. Some other benefits of self-acceptance include: a sense of freedom, a decrease in fear of failure, an increase in self-worth and self-esteem, no desire to win the approval of others, kindness to ourselves when mistakes happen, a desire to live for ourselves and not for others, the ability to take risks openly regardless of the opinions of naysayers, and the ability to maintain healthy relationships with others.

A story called "A Man Named Bad"[18] really solidified for me that we are just souls inside of vessels, and that our outside can't define the inside. It's a little deep, but really read it, then re-read it and see if it hits you like it hit me.

*There once was a teacher in India who led his students in sacred teachings. One of these students was named Bad; he didn't like his name and found it sounded disgraceful and unlucky. He asked his teacher for a new, more pleasant name that would bring good fortune rather than bad. The teacher told him to go, find the new name, and come back to change it. Bad left the city to find his new name. In a near village, a man had just died and Bad asked what his name was. People said, "His name was Alive."*

*"Alive also died?" asked Bad.*

*The people answered, "Whether his name be Alive or whether it be Dead, in either case, he must die. A name is merely a word used to recognize a person."*

*He then came across a debt-slave girl who was being beaten by her masters in the street. He asked, "Why is she being beaten?"*

*He was told, "Because she is a slave until she pays back her loan debt. She returned with no money." "And what is her name?" he asked.*

*"Her name is Rich," they said.*

*"By her name she is Rich, but she has no money?" asked Bad.*

*They said, "Whether her name be Rich or Poor, in either case, she has no money. A name is merely a word used to recognize a person."*

*Completely satisfied with his own name, Bad returned home.*

*"Have you found a good name?"*

*He answered, "Sir, those named Alive and Dead both die, and Rich and Poor may be penniless. Now I know that a name is merely a word used to recognize a person. So I'm satisfied with my name."*

*By seeing Alive as dead, Rich as poor, Bad had accepted himself.*

How can we find self-acceptance? There is no quick fix or twelve step guide, and we sure as hell won't arrive at a place of self-acceptance overnight. It takes extensive work and dedication. But learning how to love, and treat yourself right can impact the way you live your life and the things you're able to accomplish. In what ways can we begin our journey of self-acceptance?

**Be kind to yourself.** It's time to accept the fact that no one judges you more than you judge yourself. You can be your own worst enemy, so you need to get out of your way and start developing patience, especially with yourself. Be gentle with yourself and accept yourself — your strengths, your areas of growth, and any challenges you face.

**Confront your fears.** We all have a past that might be filled with some not-so-great experiences in it. Let's face it, we are human, we all have some kind of baggage full of hurt and pain that we carry around with us — sometimes consciously, other times subconsciously. This baggage in turn impacts our daily lives — the way we interact with others, how we approach situations, and the choices we make. As humans, we crave and do best with routine; often we are afraid to experience new things and take on new ventures, so we get trapped in the play-it-safe-stick-to-what's-familiar bubble. Write a list of fears and then take the time to confront them head on. Have a fear-to-do list and start taking your power back!

**Use the power of positivity.** Surround yourself with goodness. Write yourself love notes. Tell yourself positive things to lift yourself up. When you feel insecurity and doubt creeping up in your thoughts, combat them by using more positive energy and thinking. Tell that Negative Nelly in your head to beat it!

**Remember: Progress, not perfection.** Let go of the ideals you see floating around in society. Let go of what you think perfection *should* look like. Don't let an obsession for perfection slow you down in accomplishing your goals. Good is good enough. And you, my dear friend, are more than enough.

**Don't take it personally.** If something offends you, stop and ask yourself why you're offended. Oftentimes, when we take a step back to examine *why* something triggered us or brought certain feelings to the surface, we will come face-to-face with certain aspects of ourselves that we haven't yet had our chance to make peace with or heal from fully. This brings me to my next point . . .

**Forgive.** Forgive others for things they didn't mean to do. Forgive yourself for mistakes you think you've made.

**Believe in yourself.** You can do anything you set your mind to. Great things can come when you believe that you can do anything, because you can. You are a strong woman and can deal with any challenge that comes your way. A great way to remind yourself of this is to keep a list of all of the cool things you proved you could do in the past, to look back on when feeling down and know you are pretty da bomb!

**Never give up!** When you fall, you need to get up and keep going. We need to forget the negative connotation surrounding the word *failure*. Instead of feeling dejected or being overly critical of ourselves every time things don't go your way, try channeling that energy into finding another way, another path to achieve your goal.

The ability or inability to accept yourself directly affects the quality of your relationships, your work, your family, your free time, your decisions, and your future. So self-acceptance isn't just crucial to get the body you always wanted . . . It is needed in all facets of life!

## SELF-LOVE

Self-love is a regard for one's own happiness and advantage (chiefly considered as a desirable rather than narcissistic characteristic).[19] It seems like everyone is on a quest to find self-love, but how do we find it? (Order it off Amazon.com? We wish!) Here is my brief guide on how to start loving yourself:

**Begin your day with love (not technology).** Instead of reaching for your gadget and scrolling through your social media feeds first thing in the morning, begin each new day with positive and empowering thoughts about yourself.

**Take time to meditate and journal.** These introspective activities can give your mind and heart a sense of calm and direction, and they also act as an incubator for creative ideas or ventures. You really do discover your deepest longings and thoughts when you take the time to meditate and journal daily.

**Train your mind with positive affirmations.** The words you speak to yourself are just as powerful as the thoughts you think. It is easy to fall into a negative thought spiral; however, we can train our mind to see the good in almost every situation and approach life with an empowered mindset by having our thoughts, words, and actions match up. Utilize positive affirmations, intentions, or whatever works for you to view things in an empowering and positive light and seize control of your life.

**Continue to learn and be curious.** Take up a new hobby. Try something new. Learn a language. Take a trip. Feed your mind, body, and soul with new experiences. Warning: You might just find yourself in the process.

**Enjoy life more.** Spend more time with friends or those who lift you up. Do things you love. Volunteer for a cause you believe in. Start that business you've always wanted to start. Have some fun. Life's too short to make it all work and no play!

**Surrender to what you can't control.** Like the song from the movie *Frozen — LET IT GO*. Breathe, relax, and stop trying to find answers or justifications. What will be, will be.

**Work on spiritual development.** We are here to learn and love on a deeper level. Challenge yourself to find newer levels of understanding, both of yourself and of those around you, to live with intention, and to approach things from a place of love and kindness.

**Own your potential.** Love yourself enough to believe that you are limitless and that all things are possible for you if you believe in yourself and your talents, abilities, and gifts.

**Be patient with yourself.** Don't rush — take the time you need to be your best.

**Appreciate yourself.** Love all your flaws and imperfections. They are what make you, you!

**Trust your instincts.** That feeling you get in the pit of your stomach is always right. Always listen to your inner voice — that is your instinct.

**If it's toxic, it has to go.** Don't allow people who are toxic or negative to have a place in your life. Be picky with whom you spend your precious time.

**Be present.** The past is the past. You cannot change it, but you can learn from it and lead a more present and intentional life because of those past experiences.

**Forgive yourself.** Learn from your mistakes and move forward. You are doing your best.

**Be real.** Stop pretending to be someone you're not. Drop the facade and be your true self. Playing a fake role is draining, exhausting, and takes away from the love we can give to ourselves.

**Focus on the positive.** In almost every situation, there can be a silver lining — find it.

**Stand strong in your beliefs.** Don't allow anyone to change your views or your mission.

**Believe in your own self-worth.** You are worthy of love and so much more. Once you believe that wholeheartedly, self-love will start flowing freely.

## SELF-ESTEEM

Self-esteem reflects an individual's confidence and satisfaction in oneself.[20] It is the attitude and belief that people hold toward themselves. Synonyms of self-esteem and related concepts include: self-worth, self-regard, self-respect, and self-integrity. People with a healthy level of self esteem:

- Firmly believe in certain values and principles and are ready to defend them even when they face opposition; they also feel secure enough to modify their principles in light of experience.

- Are able to act according to what they think to be the best choice, trusting their own judgment and not feeling guilty when others do not like their choice.

- Do not lose time worrying excessively about what happened in the past or about what could happen in the future. They learn from the past and plan for the future, but live in the present intensely.

- Fully trust in their capacity to solve problems, not hesitating after failures and difficulties. They ask others for help when they need it.

- Consider themselves equal in dignity to others, rather than inferior or superior, while accepting differences in certain talents, personal prestige, or financial standing.

- Understand that they are an interesting and valuable person.

- Resist manipulation and collaborate with others only if it seems appropriate and aligned.

- Admit and accept different internal feelings and drives, either positive or negative, and reveal those drives to others only when they choose.

- Are able to enjoy a great variety of activities.

- Are sensitive to the feelings and needs of others; respect generally accepted social rules and claim no right or desire to prosper at others' expense.

- Can work toward finding solutions and voice discontent without belittling themselves or others when challenges arise.

So, how can we increase our self-esteem and sustain it despite what life throws our way? Here are some easy ways:

**Focus on your positive traits.** When you wake up in the morning and head to the mirror, don't pick yourself apart to find flaws. Concentrate on the things that make you beautiful and unique, like your beautiful eyes or that killer smile of yours. Try making a list of your accomplishments, rather than dwelling on your failures.

**Say goodbye to negative self-talk.** Quit beating yourself up when things don't go as planned, kicking yourself when you're down, or always telling yourself that you are not good enough. Stop telling yourself how you *should* be, and allow yourself the freedom to just be.

**Accept your feelings for what they are, without internalizing them.** Recognize that your negative feelings or the negative stories you tell to and about yourself are not the truth.

**Take action every day.** Practice makes perfect. Every day, make sure you engage in behaviors and activities that light you up. This will boost your self-confidence, self-love, hence raising your self-esteem.

**Smile so brightly.** People who smile feel happier and better about themselves. Smiling boosts confidence and just helps your self-esteem soar. So let me see those pearly whites!

Now that you have mastered self-acceptance, self-love, and self-esteem . . . learn to incorporate self-care.

## SELF-CARE

Self care means any activity that we do deliberately in order to take care of our mental, emotional, and physical health.[21] Although it's a simple concept in theory, it's something we overlook quite often. Good self-care is key to improving your mood and reducing your anxiety levels. It's also key to having a good relationship with yourself and others. Although self-care means different things to different people, here are some excellent ideas to get us on our way:

**Compliment yourself often.** Write compliments down so you can refer back to them. Better yet, leave random love notes to yourself all over your house. It'll make you smile, and give you an immediate boost of confidence.

**Take time to just sit back, relax, and smell the roses.** Take nice strolls, meditate, or even take a chill bubble bath.

**Stop taking the little things for granted.** Don't rush through your daily drive or the daily dog walk, making yourself coffee, or even a warm shower. Instead, enjoy the moment you are in.

**Laugh often.** They say laughter is the best medicine, and rightfully so. Just as smiling helps with self-love, use laughter for self-care.

**Be selfish. Put yourself first for a change.** Do one thing today just because it makes you happy.

**Put the gadgets away.** Do a technology cleanse for a short time each day. This will help you tune into your own life more and be present and mindful.

**Unfollow, block, or delete — online as well as IRL (in real life).** Just like we did in chapter three with our social media accounts, remove the negative energy and draining people from your real life.

**Learn to breathe.** Use meditation, yoga, or just mindfully focusing on the breath.

**Dance like everyone's watching.** It can feed your self-care to just dance and bounce around.

**Take a moment to stretch.** This can mean simply standing up and reaching for the sky, or doing full-fledged stretches that help loosen stiff muscles and release stress at the same time.

**Get naked.** No, not for sex (although that works, too). In all seriousness, bare it all and look at your body - all of it, with full acceptance and love for every curve and edge.

**Hydrate, hydrate, hydrate.** Drinking eight to twelve glasses of water a day will do wonders for your health — inside and out.

**Get outside and load up on Vitamin D**. Soak up the sunshine and find as much nature as you can to feed your soul and take care of your overall well being.

**Take a cat nap.** Naps are amazing and do wonders to rejuvenate the mind and body. Whether you have a busy, jam-packed day or not, take a power nap or a cat nap. Just try it even once. It's amazing what fifteen to twenty minutes of sleep can do for your well-being

**Be kind to yourself. Be your own best friend first.** Treat yourself like you treat your best friend, and use positive self-talk to support this.

**Listen to uplifting recordings or podcasts on the drive to work.** Turn a negative, traffic-packed commute into a time to listen to positive self-help books, uplifting biographies, etc.

**Help a stranger. Give the gift of kindness to someone who needs it.** Help someone carry groceries to their car, compliment the clerk at the grocery store on her haircut, or just say good morning to someone with a smile. Lift others up to internally care for yourself.

**Date yourself. Learn to fill your cup by enjoying your own company.** Spend an hour alone doing something that nourishes you (reading, practicing a hobby, visiting a museum or gallery, etc.). Time alone is the most valuable thing you can give yourself in terms of self-care. It helps you become more self-aware, confident, self-assured, and empowered.

So there you have it — master the four S's to help you on your journey to rocking the shit out of your body! Start with just two or three things off each of the lists to begin the inner work and healing, and watch the outsides follow.

*We all have problem areas. I'm always going to have thick thighs. I can't change that, and obsessing over it will only make me miserable. Learning to be grateful for our bodies and taking care of them are the best ways for us to empower ourselves physically, mentally, and spiritually.*

~ DEMI LOVATO

💋 **ROCK WITH US**

Write a list of what you do for self-care now, and what you'd like that list to look like below. Then take a photo of you doing something from the "wish" list every time you add it to your routine, and send your pic to **#kissmycurvyassets**!

NOW                                    TO ADD

_____        _____

_____        _____

_____        _____

_____        _____

_____        _____

## NOTES

_____

_____

_____

_____

_____

_____

_____

_____

_____

_____

_____

_____

## NOTES

---

# CHAPTER 9

# ACHIEVE THE THREE M'S (MEDITATION, MANTRAS, MOTIVATION)

*It's something that's with you for your whole life. You learn your mantra, it never leaves you, and it's the deepest rest your brain gets. For people that are so creative and have this kind of creative faucet that never turns off – it just continues and continues – it can be a little exhausting. And, you know, with the continual responsibility of having 127 people on the road, and always being the point person for everything, my subconscious is going even when I'm sleeping. I'm dreaming about whatever I'm creating next, or relationships, or blah, blah, blah. So I'm never really off. And meditation is actually the one time I get to really reset.*

~ KATY PERRY

We keep talking about this concept of mastering the internal so that the external can follow. But what does that really mean? How can we find a deeper connection to ourselves? That doesn't necessarily mean sitting in a corner chatting with the Dalai Lama… although that would be freakin' cool! What if there were three easy techniques or ways to help us to just switch our focus to the internal, so that those outside goals automatically followed suit? No pressure, no forcing those goals. Just smooth, seamless killin' it and smashing those external goals because we have finally mastered how to focus on our inner goddess.

## MEDITATION

My first thought when I used to hear this word: *Run! Run fast! Run far, far away! Seriously, Lori, runnnn!* I would sigh and insert the world's largest eye roll! I was *that* girl in yoga class, the one who would start a mental marathon of running through my to-do list and grocery list during the meditation sequence in class. Or I would look around to see how crazy the rest of the class looked sitting so still, not moving or thinking. Or I would just fall asleep and be snoring during it!

A former fitness mentor of mine, Barb, tells a story about when she went to India to study yoga and meditation. Her teacher would make them sit in the heat, crossed-legged and eyes closed, unable to move at all, for hours and hours. She remembers bugs landing on her and not being able to swipe them away. She remembers a time when she was trying so hard to calm her mind but could feel a drizzle of sweat on the tip of her nose, just ready to drip down. Oh, how she wanted to wipe it away! But she was training her mind, unable to move.

Now, I am not talking about meditating to this deep extent (I would have been *that* badass to just wipe the sweat away and call it a day), but I am suggesting small amounts of time to be still, to calm your mind from its endless chatter. I used to think my yoga mentors were crazy when they would tell me to meditate for five to twenty minutes a day. I kept thinking, *Me? You want someone like me, who is so high-strung, energetic, and so full of it, to sit still and calm my mind?! You've gotta be kidding me! You must be crazy!* BUT... when we do take time to meditate, the mental, emotional, and physical benefits are phenomenal. Meditation is a powerful tool that helps reduce stress, boost our physical health, ease chronic pain, and support better sleep. Meditation has also been proven to improve mental and emotional well-being in the long term. On a deeper level, meditation can also help open us to the cosmic universe (or spiritual consciousness) that is within each of us. (Okay, easy there, Lori! That got a little too spiritual, even for me.)

Remember, folks, a little bit goes a long way!! We don't need to sit still for hours, with bugs flying all around us and beads of sweat trickling down our nose. Meditation is like a muscle that grows stronger the more you use it. Like me, you might spend the first few times moving around, feeling a bit uncomfortable, opening your eyes every few seconds, mentally running through grocery or to-do lists, or just unable to clear your mind. But keep practicing! If you've never tried to meditate, don't worry. It's incredibly simple to start:

1. Find a quiet spot where you will not be interrupted or distracted.

2. Sit or lie down in a comfortable position. Feel free to use pillows to make your experience more enjoyable.

3. Make no effort to control your breath — simply breathe normally.

4. Bring your attention to your breath. In and out. In and out.

5. Bring your attention to your body and thoughts.

6. Bring your attention to any emotions that are present.

7. Be kind to yourself. There is no right or wrong way to meditate.

Wherever your mind wanders, it's okay. Simply guide your mental focus back to your breath. Whatever emotions come up, simply be with them. Some people feel physical energy moving through their body, and others feel sadness, anger, or even laughter come through. The key is to be kind and gentle with yourself. Start in small increments and work up to more time as you become more used to it. A good beginning goal is two to five minutes. Set a timer so you don't have to wonder about an end time. If you use your phone as a timer, make sure to mute all text, phone call, and social media notifications, or they can be quite distracting.

Want an even easier way to meditate? The beautiful power of technology! There are some amazing guided meditation apps, such as Headspace. It is SO GOOD! And it's easy to use!

## MANTRAS

There is no generally accepted definition of a mantra. Some define it as a thought, prayer, or even a super power. Many think of it as a verbal way to get something into one's mind. *The Oxford Living Dictionary* defines a mantra as: A word or sound repeated to aid concentration in meditation. *The Cambridge Dictionary* provides two different definitions. The first refers to Hinduism and Buddhism: A word, short phrase, or sound that is believed to have a special spiritual power. The second definition is more general: A word or phrase that is often repeated and expresses a particularly strong belief.

There are no rules when choosing your mantras. They can be simple and unique to you. We can often combine meditation and mantras, repeating the mantra during our short meditations to keep the mind focused or calm. I also love printing off my mantras and framing them so I can view them each day.

Here are some of my personal favorites that you can use as inspiration. Find something that resonates with you, makes you feel something, and fits with your real life and feelings.

# ACHIEVE THE THREE M'S...

~ Choose purpose over perfect.

~ Yesterday is not today.

~ Just ride this wave.

~ Inhale the future, exhale the past.

~ Be a warrior, not a worrier.

~ Everything I need is within me.

~ Let go of the what ifs.

~ Life is short, smile while you still have teeth.

~ Confidence is something you create within yourself by believing in who you are.

~ I love myself, I believe in myself, I support myself.

~ Don't give up what you want the most for what you want right now.

~ Positive mind, positive life.

~ What's meant to be will always find a way.

~ I am present now.

~ Be with those who bring out the best in you, not the stress in you.

~ Life doesn't get easier, you just get stronger.

~ I give myself permission to slow down.

~ I am free from sadness.

~ Expect nothing and appreciate everything.

~ Be in love with your life, every minute of it.

Remember to find your own words or phrases that call out to you, work with you, and hit close to your mind and heart. A tip I love and have used with clients and myself is to write the mantra on my washroom mirror with lipstick or washable marker, so when I get out of the shower, brush my teeth, or when I'm doing my makeup, I am reminded of it! The mantra I used on my mirror when writing this book was "You are one kick ass babe!" (Hey, whatever works!)

## MOTIVATION

*The Oxford Dictionary* defines motivation as 1) the general desire or willingness of someone to do something, and 2) a reason or reasons for acting or behaving in a particular way.

Sometimes you propel yourself out of bed in the morning and head to the gym, but other times you hit snooze. Sometimes you pick the better foods that help you get to your fitness goals, but other times you throw in the towel and drink the wine. Without motivation, daily tasks become tougher and reaching your fitness goals or body ideals almost impossible.

What habits can we use to kick ourselves in the ass(ets) and get on track towards our fitness goals?

**Start small, and go steady.** Don't focus on gung-ho big leaps that make you want to procrastinate. If a project or task feels too big and daunting, it can make you feel overwhelmed and stuck in action-paralysis. Instead, break it down into small steps and then take just one of those steps to start moving forward. Focus on baby steps toward your fitness goals instead of giant leaps.

**Reduce the daily distractions.** When you have easily accessible distractions all around you, it becomes hard to focus. So when you are at the gym, put the phone away. Don't fall into the trap of just looking at social media notifications "just for a second" — this often turns into wasted time away taken from your precious workout.

**Get accountability from the people in your life.** Find a training partner or just a text buddy to remind one another to get to the gym. This accountability partner can also encourage you to get back out there when you fall back into old mindsets and negativity.

**Get motivation from the people in your life.** Spend less time with negative people who always look at the dark side of things, and spend more of the time you have with enthusiastic or motivated people and let their energy flow over to you. This tip rings especially true for social media. Unfollow or block the "Debbie Downers" and those who strip you of motivation and make you feel terrible.

**Play music that gives you energy.** One of the simplest things I do when I feel demotivated or have low energy is to play music that is upbeat and / or inspires me. For me, a good 90s dance party will help kick my butt in the gym and just gets me working harder, thus producing results! (Who isn't motivated with "Mr. Vain" or "Rhythm is a Dancer" on full blast during a sweat session?)

**Find the optimism.** Pessimism can drain both your motivation and your energy. A positive and constructive way of looking at things, on the other hand, can energize and recharge your motivation. So when you're in what looks like a negative situation, ask yourself, "What's one thing that's good about this?" For example, maybe you missed your workout, BUT instead you went for a nice long walk with a friend.

**Be kind to yourself when you stumble.** It's so easy to fall into the trap of beating yourself when you stumble. So try this the next time — be kind to yourself, just get back on track, and keep taking small steps forward.

**Compare yourself to yourself and see how far you have come.** Instead of deflating yourself and your motivation by comparing yourself to others who don't have the same real-life as you, look back at old pics or workout logs, and see how far you have come.

**Remind yourself of why you are working toward this.** When you're feeling unmotivated and low in energy, it's easy to lose sight of why you're doing something. So take two minutes and write down your top three reasons for eating healthy and working out. Come back to that whenever you want to skip a workout or eat the whole pizza.

**Remind yourself of what you're moving away from.** You can also motivate yourself to get going again by looking at the negative impact of your current path. Ask yourself, "Do I really want to keep harming my body with this up and down extreme mentality? Will this spiral me back into the same old habits I am fighting so hard to leave behind?"

**Mix things up.** A rut will kill motivation, so mix things up. Try new foods, pull out some recipes you haven't made in a while, or revamp your workout regimen. Try that new trail you've been wanting to explore. Join that running group or soccer team.

**Adjust your goal size.** If a big fitness goal feels overwhelming, set a smaller goal to find your motivation again. It's the smaller goals that will eventually help you reach your bigger goal anyway.

**Reward yourself and celebrate your successes (no matter how big or small).** Look forward to and treat yourself to a nice reward after you have hit fitness milestones. This doesn't have to centre around food alone. Maybe a spa day with girlfriends or a shopping trip for some new clothes!

**Take a two-minute meditation break.** It'll calm the nerves and curb your stress levels.

**Go out in nature.** When you are about to eat something that doesn't support your fitness goals, why not head for the hills? Get some fresh air and head for a relaxing or powerful walk to clear your mind. This not only sidetracks you from giving in to temptation, it also allows you to smell the fresh air and take a moment to just be.

Remember the three M's — meditation, mantras, and motivation — not only when it pertains to your health and fitness goals but also when you're trying to let go of caring what society thinks and rock the shit out of your body. Use these tools to focus on yourself and what you want. Remember — focus on the internal, and the external goals will happen naturally!

*Step away from the mean girls and say bye-bye to feeling bad about your body and your looks. Are you ready to stop colluding with a culture that makes so many of us feel physically inadequate? Say goodbye to your inner critic, and take this pledge to be kinder to yourself and others.*

~ OPRAH

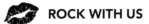
## ROCK WITH US

Write a mantra on your bathroom mirror for the week and take a pic. Hashtag **#kissmycurvyassets** so we can see what you are using for weekly/daily inspiration.

## NOTES

# CHAPTER 10

# GET NAKED FREQUENTLY - ORGASM OFTEN!

*Make sure he knows you're entitled to an orgasm. I like to say it. I'll be like - "Have you met my clit?"*

~ AMY SCHUMER

There is nothing more powerful than the female orgasm. Nothing more amazing than your body reaching that full climax, when every inch of you is quivering and you're unable to speak. Nothing better than feeling fierce, sexy, feminine, wild, and most of all, feeling free and uninhibited!

Holla - do I have your attention?

Imagine accepting your body for all its beauty, glory, and every single detail - every curve, edge, jiggle, bump, lump, imperfection. Imagine allowing yourself to feel like a SEX GODDESS. Imagine if you had no hang-ups about your body and could just "get off" without worrying about how you look mid-act or what your partner may be thinking.

In all my life, through so many female friendships, no matter what their size or body fat percentage, have I ever heard a woman say that a man didn't want to have sex with her because of the extra ten pounds she was carrying. In fact, society (and rap music videos) will show us that the more junk there is in the trunk, the more to grab on to, the more cushion-for-the-pushin, the more intense an orgasm is for a man. Ladies, I'll let you in on another big secret — being voluptuous, healthy, curvy, and, more importantly, being confident and rocking the shit out of your body is the ultimate turn-on!

Women's bodies are a turn-on, no matter what the size. A woman who is in tune with her own sexuality is hot AF. A woman who walks the walk and talks the talk of a sex goddess can rule the world (and given the state of the current political union, it could be something to consider!). So have more sex, and orgasm like you have never orgasmed before. Do it again, and again! Just get naked!

Now here is some homework I want to do! More sex! More orgasms! More time naked! How amazing will it feel to embrace and finally rock the shit out of our bodies? But is it really that easy?

This is my favorite chapter (lots of research needed for this one!), as female sexuality and female pleasure are just not talked about often enough or candidly enough. Men are allowed to brag about getting off constantly, but thanks to the social taboo still permeating women's sexuality (pfft, double standards, honestly), women tend to keep their sexuality more secretive. Why is this the case? And better yet — why is sex such an important part of learning to embrace and rock your body? Besides the obvious answer of learning to tune into your sexual energy, there are also some other health benefits from achieving the Big O:

**More sex = less stress**. And less stress means your adrenal glands are not fatigued and your hormones are balanced and stable = weight loss. Pleasurable behaviors, like having sex and eating high-calorie comfort foods, reduce stress via our brain reward pathways, according to research published in the Proceedings of the National Academy of Sciences of the United States of America.[22]

**Heart health.** More sex = more heart pumping = less chance of heart disease. Now this is cardio you can sign me up for!

**Sleep better.** Ever have the best orgasm of your life and then roll over and have the best sleep of your life? An intense orgasm releases prolactin, oxytocin, and endorphins. All of these hormones produce a sedative-like effect on the body.

**Prevent prostate cancer.** The orgasm that your male partner or spouse is having will aid in the prevention of prostate cancer. This is obviously great news for him, but let's be selfish here for a second — that also means he will live longer and can then ensure that YOU have more orgasms! The magic number is at least twenty-one orgasms for your male partner per month[23] - so get going, ladies, that's almost daily!

**Boost immune system.** Being sick less often = not missing exercise = better quality of daily life = fitness goals! Research has also shown that swapping juices during a make-out session gives you different strains of bacteria, hence strengthening your immune system even more and helping your body to be better equipped to tackle infections.[24]

**Be more youthful.** Having the Big O may also be the key to turning back the clock. Dr. David Weeks, a British clinical psychologist, spent ten years questioning thousands of men and women between the ages forty and fifty about their sexual practices as time went on. The ones who looked the youngest after a decade reported having sex thrice a week, as opposed to their not-so-youthful counterparts who had sex twice a week. Weeks says, "Sexual satisfaction is a major contributor to quality of life, ranking at least as high as spiritual or religious commitment and other morale factors, so more positive attitudes towards mature sex should be vigorously promoted." Have more sex to live longer? Sign me up!

**We can't forget the obvious. Orgasm more = be happier!** Release those endorphins time after time with a really good, body-shaking orgasm, and you are sure to skip around like Little Bo Peep the rest of the day!

Okay, so sex, or orgasms might not replace your daily workout at the gym — or can it?? Let's talk about calories burned during some sexual activities:[25]

**Kissing: 68 calories burned per hour.** I get chills thinking about that one amazing kisser. You know. The kiss that you just never wanted to end. You could almost orgasm just from locking lips. "If the kissing is vigorous and involves some petting, it could be even closer to 90 calories burned in an hour," says Jaiya Kinzbach, a Los Angeles–based sexologist and the author of *Red Hot Touch.*

**Having sex: 144+ calories burned per half-hour.** Ever have such an intense, sweaty session that it reminded you of that double spin class you decided to take that one time? Reap the extra benefits of actually orgasming in the end, and just take the sex instead! Experts say the key to high-calorie-burning sex is making it hot and making it last. Plus, almost, but not quite, having the big O over and over again will bring you to the most intense one yet — build-up is a good thing. So tease away, almost climax, and then keep going! Try positions that involve squatting, grinding on top, standing and from behind . . . whew, it is hot in here!? Perhaps the best way to maximize calorie-burning during sex is to make sure you orgasm. Experts estimate that women who orgasm during sex burn more calories during lovemaking than those who don't. So don't leave that session without achieving your end goal!

**Giving oral sex: 100 calories burned per half-hour.** Now, we don't want our partner to think we need them for our workout, but think about this. You can pleasure your partner AND burn off the chocolate you indulged in after dinner. Score!

**Who wants a hand job? 100 calories burned per hour.** Try really slow, sensual strokes, and position yourself so that you can use your body as well.

**Making Out: 238 calories burned per half-hour.** An intense make-out session may also be the most intense calorie blaster. More build-up! Your heart is racing, you are breathing heavily, rolling around and burning tons of calories. Turn up the heat in the room for even more of a calorie burn — think "Bikram yoga," but naked and with an orgasm at the end!

So, if I do the math correctly, on any given evening, I could burn around 700 calories!

| ACTIVITY | BURNED |
|---|---|
| Say, some light kissing for a half hour | 70 CALS |
| Then some hot-and-heavy making out for a half hour for more anticipation | 238 CALS |
| Follow it up by a little hand job, little oral for your partner | 150 CALS |
| Then some crazy intense sex with numerous positions for a half hour (intense I said!) | 200 CALS |
| **SUBTOTAL** | **658 CALS** |
| Add that insane orgasm at the end, combined with some build-up, and it's sure to put us closer to 1000 total calories burned! | |
| **GRAND TOTAL CALORIES BURNER** | **1000+ CALS** |

Whew! I am canceling my gym membership! SOLD!

Okay, I will state the obvious — this works well with a partner, but what do we do if we are single and solo? You orgasm on your own! It's totally normal for people to talk about guys jerking off, but there's this cultural stigma around women and masturbation. Why do we have such a hard time talking about playing with ourselves? There is nothing to be embarrassed about! We need it just like we need sleep, food, and to brush our teeth! Earlier on, we talked about the benefits of intense sex with a partner, masturbating can actually help you figure out what works for you so you can share it with your partner.

Masturbating can actually also help us as women feel better about our bodies and our sexuality. Sure, we know pleasuring ourselves reduces stress, helps us sleep, makes us happy, clears our head, gives us energy, and helps our immune system, but let's talk about the self-confidence it gives us. When you take control of how you feel about your body, your sexuality, your naked self, you feel even more fierce, empowered, and sexy.

Remember the movie *Bridget Jones Diary*: "Bridget Jones, wanton sex goddess, with every bad man between her thighs." You see, Bridget didn't have this model body, she wasn't super lean or trim, but she accepted her body and was a sex goddess in bed. And look who she landed — hottie Hugh Grant! When you reclaim your power over your sexuality, you can then ask for what you want when you are in bed with a partner. You know what gets you off, you know what feels good, you know what you need to quiver like never before!

Another benefit of playing with yourself often is increasing your libido — the more you do it, the more you want it! Pleasuring yourself can help rev up your libido, and your relationship with a partner, whereas hormones, daily stressors, and other factors can impact and decrease libido. Fingers, rabbits, dildos, vibrators, let's not get picky here . . . the options are endless. Lose the fear and head to your local sex toy shop, or heck, purchase online! Ask your girlfriends about their favorite sex toys. Let's stop being so afraid to talk about our sexuality!

So all of this sex talk has me unable to think perfectly clear, and it sure sounds easy. But how do we become comfortable in our own skin, accepting every part of our self? Guess what? Practice makes perfect. Here are some really easy ways to feel better when totally in the flesh:

**Be realistic.** Remember that the media is playing with our minds, with all of the air brushing, etc. Just look at the porn industry. I mean seriously, do we really look and sound like that during sex? Stop comparing yourself to others, and find love for your body. Look at yourself naked and write down everything you love about your body. You do you, naked!

**Practice. Yes, be naked.** Growing up, I had a friend from Brazil, or somewhere where nudity was no biggie. Her mother would prance around the house in her birthday suit. Totally naked. Sometimes she would be in her bra and short shorts, but usually she was just happy putting it all out there. She was comfortable in her own skin. Her children were the same way. They never felt the need to hide, or nor did they feel ashamed about their bodies, breasts, or butts. I had one girlfriend in college who slept naked, walked to the shower in the co-ed dorm naked, had full conversations with you while eating Kraft dinner, naked. When I was around her, I also felt liberated to just be naked. I was more open to realizing that it was just a body, and that to be comfortable in it felt so good. It's amazing how good it can feel to just walk around naked. It might be asking a lot for you to start walking through the grocery stores naked (and you might get arrested). But next time you are home alone, wander around naked. Do the dishes naked, vacuum the house naked (although that reminds me of a famous *Seinfeld* episode, in which they determine that not everything looks good when done naked!). Just be with yourself, naked. Walk past mirrors, see how wonderful it is to just roam free.

**Masturbate with mirrors.** When you pleasure yourself, have mirrors everywhere. Keep your eyes open and the lights on. Experience what it is like to be with yourself naked! Wow, is your partner or future partner ever lucky to have such a sex goddess like you! How does it feel to actually see yourself in the flesh!? Even better? Record yourself while you do it and then watch it later, or even better, save it and let your partner watch it later for an even more intense arousal. (Just put a darn lock or password on your phone people, this dang technology always backfires on us later!). There is also something to be said for a good old-fashioned sex tape. How empowering does it feel to watch yourself in action? See how amazing your body is, and even better, see how excited your partner feels to be with such an amazing being as you.

Getting comfortable being naked is really about becoming more comfortable with yourself. It's not about oozing sex like you see in porn; it's about loving and accepting yourself and celebrating who you are as a person. Once we learn to actually see ourselves for the sex vixens we are, we can build better sex lives, have more intense orgasms, and achieve the focus of this book, which is to embrace and rock the shit out of your body. So get to your homework — sex, juices, cumming, and just feeling so comfortable in the skin you are in. 'Cause we are all porn stars in our own right, so we need to own the shit out of what we have!

*I would only lose weight if it affected my health or my sex life, which it doesn't.*

~ ADELE

---

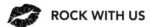 **ROCK WITH US**

Now this is the challenge I wanna be a part of. Hold up your number at the end of the month and take pic. No need to explain: the number alone will do. Share using hashtag **#kissmycurvyassets**

Let's get those numbers up there! We will know what you're telling us and be orgasm-proud with you!

---

## NOTES

_____

_____

_____

_____

_____

_____

_____

_____

_____

_____

_____

_____

_____

## NOTES

_____
_____
_____
_____
_____
_____
_____
_____
_____
_____
_____
_____
_____
_____
_____
_____
_____
_____
_____
_____
_____
_____
_____
_____
_____
_____

# LET SHIT GO, FOCUS ON THE FUTURE, AND DON'T DWELL ON THE PAST

*The great courageous act that we must all do, is to have the courage to step out of our history and past so that we can live our dreams.*

~ OPRAH

Once upon a time, there was a girl named Lori. She lost hundreds of thousands of dollars on a fitness studio she opened, and also lost her passion and ability to thrive. Lori also lost weight, gained weight, tried fads, and crashed and burned, only to gain it all back. One day, Lori chose to move ahead, to give up the madness of these fads, to forget the failure of the studio and loss of money and passion . . . But did she mask it all, or truly forgive and forget?

Ah, dwelling on the past. I swear, if they gave awards for this, I would be on the top of that podium every single time. But after decades of holding that shit with me and letting it drag me down, I realized it was not only giving me wrinkles (and larger botox bills!), it was also just not serving me well in terms of my attitude. You see, we replay past mistakes over and over again in our head, allowing feelings of shame and regret to shape our actions in the present. We continue to be frustrated about our past, yet also worry about the future. We hold stress in our minds and bodies, which in turn can create serious health issues and so much tension. We must stop allowing yesterday's stories to affect today's progress — letting go of the past is necessary to truly thrive today. We've all been hurt by others and by situations — it's part of life. But while the pain is often out of our control, I think it's helpful to remember that we *can* control how we respond to it, and how we let it go. Do we dwell on the past . . . or do we learn what we can and then get back to the more important task of living life and moving forward? And how in the heck do we release, let go, move on, and stop the madness of always thinking about the bad things in our past?

Through my decades of dwelling, I have come up with some ways to let that shit go:

**It's your choice to make. Own that control.** We have the choice to let it go. We can decide to stop the madness inside our heads and stop reliving the torture.

**Write that shit down.** When those old negative thoughts come up, journal it, get it on paper, acknowledge that it's there. I sometimes write it down and then burn it or tear it up (like I am taking control of it and then releasing it for good).

**Quit the blame game.** Poor you, victim Lori. Own that situation — mistakes happen, fuck-ups occur, poor choices are a part of life, own that blame, and move on! Empower yourself to learn from your mistakes.

**Be in the moment** (insert mantras here). Embrace the current day, the present moment, and there will be less time to think back to the bullshit of the past. Fill your life now with stuff that matters so that the past doesn't get to consume any more of your energy or time.

**Stop replaying it in your head.** It's such a vicious cycle to dwell, analyze, overthink, and just keep reliving past mistakes. Allow the thought to come into your head and then as you exhale your breath, let that shit go!

**Cry like a baby.** A good cry can actually melt away all the toxic feelings you might be carrying with you. So don't bottle it up, let those tears flow. Ugly cry right along with me! (Disclaimer - I am the ugliest crier out there, but at least I am not bottling that shit up!)

**Dance it out.** Yes, just like Ellen does on her talk show day after day, when you feel any old negative thoughts coming up, dance like your life depended on it. What a stress release to put on your favorite dance song and just let go! Car dance if you have to, with the music blaring in your Chevy, and that seat cushion you will be a-grindin'!

**Get in a good workout or exercise regimen.** Just moving your body will help you distract your mind and release all of that toxic energy.

**Plan for the future.** Sure, being present is great and all, but also focus on what your future brings. Plan it out. This will help you to stop dwelling on the past and to map out some ideas about what direction you want your future head towards, in a positive light and learning from past mistakes.

**Surround yourself with positive people.** When I get down or begin to think about that past negative shit, my friends are there to throw me a rope and save me from drowning in that sorrow. Laughing, wine drinking, heck even making fun of ourselves can help to lighten the situation and make it not seem to terrible.

I once read a classic Zen story of letting go:

*Two traveling monks came to a town where there was a young woman waiting to step out of her sedan chair. The rains had made deep puddles, and she couldn't step across without spoiling her silken robes. She stood there, looking very cross and impatient. She was scolding her attendants. They had nowhere to place the packages they held for her, so they couldn't help her across the puddle. The younger monk noticed the woman, said nothing, and walked by. The older monk quickly picked her up and put her on his back, transported her across the water, and put her down on the other side. She didn't thank the older monk; she just shoved him out of the way and departed. As they continued on their way, the young monk was brooding and preoccupied. After several hours, unable to hold his silence, he spoke out. "That woman back there was very selfish and rude, but you picked her up on your back and carried her! Then she didn't even thank you!" "I set the woman down hours ago," the older monk replied. "Why are you still carrying her?"*

This story just sits with me. All those past diets that didn't work. All the abuse we put ourselves through with extreme exercise. All our past relationship losses. All the past negative self-talk or body shaming. It just feels amazing to let that shit go!

Letting go doesn't mean forgetting the past — it just means not dwelling on it. What a waste of time and energy it is to constantly focus on something that cannot be undone. Like that monk still carrying the memory of the rude woman, why do we continue to carry the shame we have felt for not reaching or maintaining our fitness goals or achieving some impossible body ideal? If this sense of failure keeps us stuck in the past, we cannot be truly present in our lives, nor can we move forward into the future.

Our struggles don't define us, but they can help us grow. Making mistakes means we are human. Turn your struggle into a story. A success story. From every great struggle, an even greater success is born. Take Oprah Winfrey, for example. You think she had it easy getting to where she is today? Oprah faced many setbacks, but she became one of the most influential women in the world by not allowing others to define her, not giving in to her self-doubts, and not throwing in the towel when the going got tough. She endured abuse, starting with one of her first reporting jobs where she was told that she was "unfit" for tv. You think Oprah had time to dwell on the past as she climbed her way to be the mogul she is today? Heck no!

When you focus on all the bad things you've been through, it's nearly impossible to recognize when you're going through something good. It's even more challenging to create something good with what you have.

So what is your story? The stories we tell ourselves and wrap our lives around can easily limit who we become, if we let them do so. The alternative is to let go of that pain and to stop dwelling on how you've been hurt, how you've hurt yourself, or how you've failed. You have the choice to let those decisions and life stories define you or to learn and grow from them and become a stronger version of yourself. It happens. We hold onto certain thoughts and feelings and replay them over and over again in our mind. Like a bad movie, we just keep watching it on repeat even though we know the ending. We become so stuck on this one particular story, and on the thoughts and feelings that go along with it, that we get stuck in a never-ending cycle — unless we choose to rise from and above it.

This victim cycle is so hard to rid ourselves of. Think of someone who keeps complaining about the same thing, like their weight, over and over; yet they keep making poor choices when it comes to their physical health and nutrition on a day-to-day basis. They expect different results from every fad and diet that they try as a quick fix, yet they do nothing to address their habits, behaviors, and patterns for long-term success.

A change is in order — it's time to rewrite your story and create your new movie reel. Take a moment to identify a repetitive story you keep telling yourself. How long have you been stuck in this story? Do you truly want to let go of this story, since it isn't serving you? Are you ready to change your mind or feelings around the story?

When a story or event in your life becomes stuck, it can be very difficult to clear the thoughts and feelings around it. It's our emotions that keep us stuck. In order to release and let go of a repetitive cycle or story and truly rise and heal, we have to approach our stories differently. We have to be open to change and consciously work on reprogramming those thoughts. This takes time, effort, and consistent practice.

Let's recap the best way to move forward and re-write your story:

1. **Write or repeat your story out loud.** Put it on paper. You gotta find your expression to start the healing process.

2. **Respect your story, then release it.** It came into your life for a reason, but now it's served its purpose. Say goodbye to it for good! (Remember *Frozen* - let it go, let it go, can't hold it back anymore! My apologies to any moms out there who will now be chanting this song for the next week with utter disgust!)

3. **Breathe.** Feel yourself releasing your story, and all the negative emotions associated with it, with each breath you take. Still your mind and heal your heart.

4. **Tell yourself: "My story does not define me. It's time to write a new one."** It's time to release any attachments to past events — those events do not define you. It is no longer serving you to hold on and dwell. It's time for you to write a new story, a better one.

5. **Now redirect your energy from the past, to the future ahead of you.** The future is bright and filled with so much promise — choose to let go of the stories that hold you back from being your best self and living your best life. Let go of what no longer serves you.

To fully embrace and rock the shit out of your body, and to finally find your long-term fitness goals, you must let go of the past! I often remind myself, "Every slip-up, mix-up, mess-up, or fuck-up is taking you in the direction you are meant to go!" Let that shit go, and focus on rocking your body right now!

*There are no regrets in life. Just lessons.*

~ JENNIFER ANISTON

---

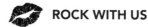 **ROCK WITH US**

Let it go: It is time to release something - anything- that you are holding onto. Write it down on a piece of paper, video yourself lighting it on fire (be fire safe) or ripping it up! Hashtag **#kissmycurvyassets** - let that shit go!

---

## NOTES

# CHAPTER 12

# ABOLISH THE GREEN-EYED MONSTER - JEALOUSY AND COMPARISON

*My body was better when I was 22, 23. But I didn't enjoy it. I was too busy comparing it to everybody else's.*

~ CINDY CRAWFORD

## *"Don't let the green-eyed monster get you."*

Do you remember hearing this saying as a kid? I actually searched for some green monster hiding in my closet for years. William Shakespeare used this saying in *The Merchant of Venice* (one of my favorites!) and *Othello* to talk about jealousy. In the context of this book, this can include being jealous of someone's ripped abs, new designer purse, hot partner, etc. I know I have been guilty of this often, and you might be able to relate.

### What is jealousy?

Jealous, or jealousy, is defined as 1) resentment against a rival, a person enjoying success or advantage, etc., or against another's success or advantage itself, 2) mental uneasiness from suspicion or fear of rivalry, unfaithfulness, etc., as in love or aims, 3) vigilance in maintaining or guarding something, or 4) a jealous feeling, disposition, state, or mood.[26]

Are you a jealous person who compares yourself to others? Does jealousy hinder your body image?

### What about comparison?

Comparison is defined as 1) the act of comparing, 2) the state of being compared, 3) a likening; illustration by similitude; comparative estimate or statement, or 4) capability of being compared or likened.[27] I honestly think I have spent most of my life trying to be someone other than myself. Always wishing I had a different body, a prettier face, nicer hair — never accepting and celebrating how unique and amazing I am, just the way I am now! All the effort and time I spent trying to to be more like everyone else only left me feeling unhappy and lost.

The truth is, it's draining to always compare ourselves to others. Aren't you tired of always striving to be something or someone you are not, and probably will never be? The comparison game can be a slippery slope, especially when we apply it to our personal fitness goals and body ideals and bring it with us when trying embrace, accept, and rock the shit out of our bodies!

I used to get so caught up in comparing myself to other women and picking apart their every flaw. Jealousy can be quite toxic — like a parasite, it feeds on all of your self-deprecating thoughts. When we surf the internet or look at images on social media, why do they trigger us and why do we internalize that as a reflection of how we feel about our bodies? I coach clients all the time who feel truly jealous of other women. We often pretend as if this behaviour is normal and acceptable, instead of saying, "This isn't right." When we feel negativity, jealousy, and envy toward other women, we are indirectly insulting ourselves. What we see in others is a reflection of what we see in ourselves. This is a normal reaction if you don't have a good body image. You see someone with something that you don't have, and you feel lousy about yourself. The problem is that when your perception of beauty is based on ridiculous ideals, you are pretty much doomed to pick yourself apart whenever you are around other women.

Remember the chapters on social media and societal ideals? Well, we get to create our own ideals. We have the power to define how we want to look and what fitness success looks like to us, in our real lives. Instead of looking at these images that would normally feed the green-eyed monster in us, we can fill ourselves with positive feelings toward these other women. The most beautiful gift you can give yourself is the ability to stop feeding the green-eyed monster, this jealousy we have of others, and this idea of perfection we keep pushing onto ourselves. The most beautiful woman that I can be is . . . ME, damn it! But in order to be fully accepting of yourself for who you truly are, you have to be willing to accept that everyone is beautiful in their own right and has their own unique strengths, traits, talents, and skill sets.

Last week, I met a friend for coffee. This is a woman who is drop-dead gorgeous and with a body I would sell my first born for. She just looks like this without effort — she wakes up looking like a supermodel. For years, I was envious, but today, I admire her. I like to celebrate her amazing body and tell her all about the things that I would have previously been jealous of. Through the years, I realized that she, too, gets jealous of other women, she, too, has her insecurities. We are all freakin human, after all.

Jealousy usually highlights what we think we are lacking. But is that just our mind playing tricks on us? Through the years of coaching thousands of women, I have often seen the comparison game played. "I wish I had ____'s abs," or "If only I had legs like _____." We are always wanting what others have, instead of looking in the mirror and admiring the amazing body and features we already have. This body we have been given is a gift in itself. Just think about it . . . we get to be here on this earth. For some of us, we get to conceive and birth children, and then raise them to be the most amazing humans and contribute to society. We have this beautiful body and soul moving around the earth capable of achieving anything we put our minds to. But are our minds clouded with so much jealousy and comparison that we stop enjoying or living life?

Let's take a moment to say this out loud . . . *it's okay to be jealous.* It's okay to have these feelings surface, so forgive yourself for feeling envious or playing the comparison game. Let's take a moment to give ourselves permission to stop this maddening competition that we have with each other as women. Let's replace competition with support for one another. Let's try collaborating and empowering each other and ourselves for a change.

Are you like me and guilty of feeling jealous around other women? What can we do to stop this madness?

**Stop the bashing.** If you have friends who engage in this behavior, don't play into it. It's a ripple effect to fall into the gossip. Make the commitment to rid your life of this wasted time and energy. Be the bigger person and seek to see the good in everyone. Remember — everyone is writing their own stories, struggling with their own battles, and living their own real lives. As women, we need to stand up for each other and end this bullshit that only magnifies our insecurities. Let's stop tearing each other down.

**Celebrate all appearances, shapes, sizes, and bodies.** Try to follow a variety of diverse people on social media. Notice the positives in other people in a non-judgmental way. We are all unique and special, and the world would be so boring if we all looked the same. Fitness comes in all shapes and sizes.

**Genuinely compliment other women.** When we say positive things to other people, we feel better about ourselves. Be genuine, and help to highlight the amazing things about other women! Your comments might be just what the doctor ordered to help them with their insecurities, jealousies, or negative feelings about themselves.

**Be grateful.** This is a super quick way to shut down jealousy. As soon as you feel that green-eyed monster creeping in, choose to be grateful for what you have instead. Being grateful for what we have often makes us forget about this comparison or "I want what she has" game we play. By choosing to be grateful and shifting our focus from a perspective of lack and envy to one of positivity and appreciation for the value we provide, we will no longer feel threatened by the wonderful things that others also have to offer. Let's be thankful for all the blessings we have in our lives instead of feeling as though we have none and are constantly lacking. The glass is always half full, my friends!

**Remember that everyone has their own struggles**. No one — no matter how "perfect" and pulled together their life or body looks on social media — is free from struggle. So you may be jealous of someone or envy them for something, but they might feel the same about you! Maybe you find yourself feeling jealous when you see a woman posting a picture on Facebook of her perfect body; you might not know that beneath that social media facade, she may be struggling with low self-worth, or she may have achieved that body through extreme dieting and training. She may be struggling with the loss of a job or with a terrible marriage. We can never fully know each other's stories, and we don't have to. We only have to accept responsibility for who we are and the choices we make each day.

**So why do we feel jealous?**

Let's talk about the "I" word . . . Insecurity.

**Insecurity** means a lack of confidence or assurance; self-doubt.[28] Body insecurities are often behind that green-eyed monster. A poll by Refinery29.com found that nearly eighty percent of the women polled said they walk around feeling somewhat dissatisfied with their bodies at least half the time. Why do our flaws hold so much power over us and how we react and respond to other women? What are you insecure about in terms of your body? Does it affect how you respond to other women? This is human nature. So how do we become more confident and rid ourselves of those insecurities?

Accept your body. Easy right!? NOT! Just when you think you are well on the road to accepting yourself and getting adjusted, life throws some new obstacle your way. What in the heck can we do to help ourselves?

**Turn a negative into a positive.** Hard as it may be, you have to take active steps to get over your insecurities and negative feelings. Insecurity breeds so many other emotions like jealousy, anger, and depression. Some things about your body cannot be changed, or perhaps they can, but only through extremes and long-term damage. For instance, a mother may hate her stomach and be insecure about it. But that same body was the one that gave life to three children. Those rolls and stretched skin served such an amazing purpose — the conception and birth of her children, the creation of life. Her body is a source of strength and feminine power. She is so blessed to have those children, and that stomach, to show how amazing she is.

**Set achievable goals with realistic expectations.** If you are insecure about your weight, it would be unrealistic to expect to lose fifty pounds in thirty days. Avoid aiming for an outcome that is unrealistic and unachievable. You may also need to choose better role models for your body ideals — are they realistic for your life?

**Seek help from a coach or professional.** Your insecurities may stem from baggage built up over decades of mental programming. With the help of a professional, you will be able to heal and undo decades worth of societal programming a lot more effectively than if you were to attempt it on your own. Sometimes hearing something from an external source can provide you with a different perspective, as it is hard to identify or be aware of a thought pattern or behavior when you're in the thick of things. You cannot heal something you are not aware of. Tackling the problem begins with recognizing that you have a negative body image in the first place and then taking conscious and consistent action to reclaim your positive self-image and esteem.

What do you think your life would look like if you could clear out the closet that green-eyed monster is lurking in it? It's time to end the game of comparisonitis and its toxic hold on us and embrace and rock the shit out of our bodies for all their glory - scars, stripes, rolls, and all! Own what you have and do so with a feminine ferocity, instead of always wondering if the grass is greener on the other side.

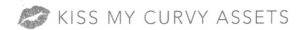 

*I don't have a Kate Moss body, but I'm very
proud and happy with mine.*

~ KATY PERRY

---

### ROCK WITH US

Write down 5 times you complimented someone else below (including
the compliment). Take a screenshot and hashtag **#kissmycurvyassets** to
share with us. We want to see you lifting others up! Share how amazing
you are being to other bad-ass babes!

WHO ROCKED | WHAT THEY ROCKED
--- | ---
_____ | _____
_____ | _____
_____ | _____
_____ | _____
_____ | _____

---

## NOTES

_____

_____

_____

_____

_____

_____

# CHAPTER 13

# IMPLEMENT NUTRITION FOR REAL LIFE

*You're only human, you only live once, and life is wonderful, so eat the damned red velvet cupcake.*

~ EMMA STONE

When I sat down to write this book, I decided that actual diet and exercise would play such a small part in it. I didn't want to write this preachy, "Eat this, not that" kind of book. There are enough books out there trying to over-complicate an already messed up subject. I wanted to keep it simple, short, and sweet. I just want you to have the tools to implement your own nutrition plan, on your own terms, for your ideal body and life. I will not provide you with a cookie-cutter diet plan that makes empty promises about fat loss and transformations. I want to educate you and provide you with the right tools so you can stop overthinking nutrition. I want you to be able to focus on *what* you are eating, *why* you choose to eat it, and of course, why you *need* it, and then see what works best for you.

While nutrition is important, it is only *one* facet in our journey of finding our ideal body and rockin' the shit out of it. Nutrition and lifestyle changes combined with emotional and mental healing will make the whole yo-yo dieting game go extinct. Instead, we will nourish our bodies and our health naturally.

A lot of women are tired of feeling frustrated, anxious, and helpless when it comes to nutrition and our bodies. Wouldn't it be so nice to have a meaningful connection with food and to be able to celebrate holidays and events without the guilt trip of "I shouldn't have eaten that?" Food is supposed to bring us energy, joy, and connection and to fuel our amazing bodies! Eating shouldn't be so complex or harsh; it should be effortless and fit into our day-to-day lives seamlessly.

There are many different ways to eat, and fuel our bodies. Finding a nutrition program that works for you and your real life is key. For example, some people choose nutrition plans that emphasize macro-nutrient and micronutrient quotients per meal, while other folks choose to focus on biofeedback such as hunger, energy, sleep, mood, and sex drive instead of emphasizing numbers, macros / micros, and restrictions. To ensure long-term success, our mindset has to shift from an "all-or-nothing" mentality to one of growth and progress. Think about food being a source of connection, a reason to gather around the table, a source that brings everyone together. Like drinking wine with girlfriends, it just *feels* good!

Over the decades, food has become less about a basic need and source of self-care and more about telling us how to feel — a reinforcement of both positive and negative emotions. If we adjust our mindsets and get rid of the "I earned it" or emotional eating mentality and focus on sustainable nutrition consistently, we can achieve those long-term fitness goals without starvation, extremes, or "yo-yo-ing". Deprivation or extreme diets often subliminally reinforce the belief that food is a prized object, a measured reward, and something with esteemed emotional value and comfort. It's much like a toddler who seeks comfort from his / her "blankie" or "stuffy" for emotional relief or reward. Reaching for food becomes a habitual way to seek positive reinforcement. It ends up being less about the actual taste and nutritional value of the food and more about the desired emotional reward. This Pavlovian response to food leads to an intense focus on food as a reward or, in some cases, a band-aid to mask emotional and mental torment. If we can reframe our perspective of food from one of "all-or-nothing mindless binging" to "conscious consumption in moderation," we can stop using food as our crutch and use it as nourishment instead.

Visualize walking down a flight of stairs. If you stumble on one step, you don't throw yourself down the whole flight of stairs. Or if your car gets one flat tire, you don't slash the other three good tires! The same goes for nutrition. If you have an off day or some slip-ups, it's best to just dust off and keep going instead of thinking, "it's all over" and continuing to go off plan. You won't gain weight from eating just one unhealthy meal, just as you won't lose weight just from eating one healthy meal!

To help women work on their relationship with food and their bodies, I came up with an acronym to help reframe our concept of nutrition:

## R.E.A.L - NUTRITION

| | |
|---|---|
| **R** | Right for your real life. |
| **E** | Easy to do without forcing. |
| **A** | Adjusted based on biofeedback (mood, energy, digestion, sex drive, etc.) |
| **L** | Loosely programmed to change as your real life changes. Not all plans can be cookie-cutter. You are unique based on genetics, dietary preferences, history, bodyweight, hormones, age, and any metabolic damage done in the past. |

You know how to nourish yourself! You have just become clouded and brainwashed by what society tells you to do and eat.

Lately we have been hearing some big buzzwords like *mindful* or *intuitive eating*, but what does this even mean?

**Mindful or Intuitive Eating is:**

- Allowing yourself to become aware of *how* your foods affect you and nurture you, and listening to your own internal voice when making food choices.

- Using all your senses to choose foods that nourish your body and also make you feel satisfied.

- Acknowledging responses to food (likes or dislikes) without judging yourself.

- Listening to your hunger cues and satiated (full) cues and using them to guide your eating decisions.

Here are some principles of this form of eating.

**Ditch the diet mentality.** Stop with the fads, trends, and labels, and be free to eat anything *you* want without these restrictions.

**Listen to your hunger cues.** That growl in your tummy is telling you something. Eat before the madness sets in or else you make poor choices out of haste. Honor your rumbling tummy by ensuring you consistently fuel your body throughout the day.

**Be friends with food.** Stop the battle with food. Stop trying to make a food "good" or "bad, "clean" or "dirty."

**Stop eating when you are full.** Listen for the body signals that tell you that you are no longer hungry. Don't get to the point of being "stuffed."

**Take pleasure in your food.** When you eat, actually *enjoy it!* Take satisfaction in the food you are so lucky to be eating. Make eating an experience rather than just going through the motions. Switch off the gadgets and sit at the table and tune out the noise around you. This helps you focus on the task at hand, which is nourishing your body with amazing fuel and nutrients.

**Think about the emotions that arise around meals and food.** If you have issues with emotional eating, search for help to resolve these issues. If you eat when you are upset, angry, anxious, or lonely, you are emotionally eating. If you find yourself raiding the pantry as soon as life throws curveballs at you, you are emotionally charged and turning to food as some fix for it. This only distracts from the pain and often numbs you in the moment, which makes things worse in the long run.

**Keep health as your top priority.** Fueling our bodies with proper foods filled with nutrients means we will live longer. Ensuring we put things into our body that aren't packed with chemicals and additives means lower risk for disease. Living a long and healthy life means using your intuition to respect your body with nutrient-packed foods, and a variety of them!.

So if we are eating mindfully, or using our intuition to fuel our nutrition choices, here are some things we could be asking ourselves before we eat to really see what our food is doing for our bodies:

- What do I hope to feel when consuming ____?

- How will eating ____make me feel?

- How will this food affect my digestion?

- How will I feel after I eat this food?

- How will my mind feel an hour after consuming ____?

- Does consuming ____support my fitness goals?

Taking the time to think about what you are about to eat, perhaps even journaling about the emotions and beliefs you have surrounding food, will help you figure out trigger situations and trigger foods. It will also highlight the foods that make you feel good and support your fitness goals.

What if we followed a plan that wasn't really a plan at all, but instead just a way of life? What does that look like?

First, let's break down the types of food out there and what they do for our bodies. *Macronutrients*, or *macros*, are proteins, fats, and carbohydrates, while *micronutrients* are vitamins, minerals, amino acids, sugars, and other nutrients. This is the basic breakdown of the food we eat. No reason to complicate it more than that. We need a variety of foods that consist of both macro and micronutrients; eliminating any of them is not a long-term solution and is just a fad and an extreme.

Here's a little more information about the different types of nutrients that we need.

## PROTEIN

This is a key nutrient that helps bind and repair tissues, build muscle, and strengthen hair, skin, and nails. Protein also helps us synthesize hormones, especially the ones that make you feel happy and relaxed. It supports our immune system, boosts our metabolism to burn more fat and keep fat off, and keeps us feeling fuller longer. You can get protein from non-vegetarian, vegetarian, and vegan sources, so there is a protein source for everyone. Non-vegetarian sources include beef, bison, pork, chicken, turkey, eggs, egg whites, and seafood like fish, scallops, and shrimp. Vegetarian and vegan sources include cheese, cottage cheese, Greek yogurt, cheese, tempeh, beans, soy, chickpeas, avocado. In addition, you can get protein from dairy-free milk and dairy-free cheese, like cashew cheese, nut milks such as almond and cashew milk, coconut milk, hemp milk, hemp seeds, etc.

## FATS

Consuming healthy sources of fat can help speed our recovery process and nourish fatty tissues such as our brain, eyes, and cells. It also helps build muscle, aids in optimal and healthy sex hormone function, improves heart and brain health, boosts memory function, and increase joint mobility. In addition, healthy fats can also improve blood lipid profile, decrease inflammation, and regulate blood sugar and metabolism. To top it all off, they decrease symptoms of depression and anxiety. Some good sources of healthy fats are oils (olive, flaxseed, coconut, avocado, and hemp), nuts and nut butters such as almonds, peanuts, hazelnuts, Brazil nuts, Macadamia nuts, and cashew nuts, seeds such as chia seeds, sunflower seeds, and pumpkin seeds, fish such as salmon, trout, and sardines, and the ever-famous avocado.

## CARBOHYDRATES

Consuming carbohydrates is essential to maintaining key bodily functions. They help regulate blood sugar, keep you fuller longer, and balance hormones due to their fiber content. There are two types of carbohydrates — complex and simple. It's common in society at large for people to satiate their appetite through simple carbohydrates such as Pop-tarts, pizza, white rice, white pasta, or bread, desserts, and other processed and refined foods. Most of the food available at fast food chains and restaurants are simple carb sources. Simple carbs do have a purpose; for example, they can provide a quick release of energy before an intense workout. But they are not an ideal long-term carb source and should be consumed more as a treat than as an everyday staple. On the other hand, complex carbohydrates are made up of a longer chain of sugars and take longer to break down in our digestive system, which is why they provide a gradual release of energy and keep us sustained for much longer without sending our blood sugar levels into overdrive. Sources of complex carbs include sweet potato, yams, yucca, amaranth, quinoa, wild rice, millet, buckwheat, kale, beans, lentils, and whole wheat bread / pasta. Did you know that vegetables are also an excellent source of fiber, complex carbs, and bioavailable vitamins? Consume a variety of vegetables (eat the rainbow!) for optimal benefits. Some of my favorites include squash, zucchini, asparagus, Brussel sprouts, cauliflower (cauliflower rice, anyone?), broccoli, spinach, kale, peppers, beets, carrots, and eggplant, just to name a few.

Here's the secret: There is no special diet to follow. It's all about eating high-quality foods, not consuming excessive calories throughout the day, and maintaining a healthy balance in the type of foods you eat.

So how does it all go together without counting calories or macros or using time-consuming apps? In a perfect world, we would have time to enter everything we ate into an app and get to see our day-to-day consumption. But let's face it — this is real life, shit happens, we are all freakin' busy! How many of us have started tracking our nutrition on an app and then after a few days or few weeks, let it slide? What if instead, we kept it super simple? Consume four meals per day with protein, carbs, and fats at each, and then have two to three snacks (around 100 calories).

Listen to your body and eat more food when needed, but make sure to nourish yourself with amazing variety. Here are a few other things to remember:

- Drink lots of water. Start your day with a warm glass of lemon water. (Why? Because the media tells us it's good for us (lol), but all kidding aside, it sets the stage for digestion.)

- Avoid getting past the point of intense hunger; try to fuel your body every two-and-a-half to three hours.

- Plan ahead and prepare some easy grab-and-go meals and snacks. Variety is the spice of life and will ensure long-term success, whereas boredom will make you want to quit and will take the enjoyment out of your fitness journey.

- Be present in your life. Allow yourself to have mental and emotional space and time when you aren't thinking about food or food prep, and are just enjoying life. Your body will tell you what to eat.

So what would this type of typical day look like nutritionally? I will give you a few samples here, and you can choose the foods you like for your meal preps. Remember, these are just examples. You need to find the food choices you like — variety is the spice of life, so mix and match and try new foods and combinations. Some people have no dietary restrictions and eat all foods, others prefer a vegetarian lifestyle, and some may be vegan. I myself am a "flexitarian." I don't really follow one set meal plan. Some days I eat fully vegan or plant-based, other days I have eggs and follow a vegetarian plan. The odd time I will also have chicken or fish. By allowing myself the flexibility of just listening to my body and eating what it is asking for without feeling like I am putting myself in XY or Z boxes. Find what works for you, and more important makes you feel amazing!

## Sample Daily Meal Plan #1 - All Foods (meat and dairy)

| | | |
|---|---|---|
| **MEAL 1** | 8:00AM | 2 whole eggs, 3 egg whites, 1/2 cup oatmeal |
| **MEAL 2** | 11:30AM | 4 oz chicken breast, 6 oz yams, mixed stir-fry veggies, 1 oz almonds |
| **MEAL 3** | 2:30PM | whey protein shake, apple with almond butter |
| **MEAL 4** | 6:00PM | 4 oz salmon, 3/4 cup wild rice, large green salad |
| Two 100-calorie snacks to be added when hungry. | | |

## Sample Daily Meal Plan #2 - Vegetarian

| | | |
|---|---|---|
| **MEAL 1** | 8:00AM | 6 egg whites, 1 tbsp flax seed oil, 6 oz nugget potatoes |
| **MEAL 2** | 11:30AM | 4 oz tofu, 1/2 cup quinoa, veggies, 1 oz cashews |
| **MEAL 3** | 2:30PM | 1 cup Greek yogurt, 2 tbsp chia seeds, 2 tbsp granola |
| **MEAL 4** | 6:00PM | 4 oz seitan or tempeh, 1/2 cup brown rice noodles, 2 tbsp tomato sauce, veggies |
| Two 100-calorie snacks to be added when hungry. | | |

**Sample Daily Meal Plan #3 - Vegan/Plant Based, Gluten Free (GF)**

| | | |
|---|---|---|
| **MEAL 1** | 8:00AM | 1 scoop plant based protein powder, 1/2 banana, 1 medjool date, ice (blend, make smoothie bowl); top with 2 tbsp homemade granola (toasted GF oats, toasted coconut, slivered almonds, hemp seeds, chia seeds) |
| **MEAL 2** | 11:30AM | 1/2 cup lentils, 1/2 cup beans, 4 oz sweet potatoes or yams, salad greens, 1 tbsp dressing of choice (goddess bowl salad) |
| **MEAL 3** | 2:30PM | 1 cup coconut yogurt, 1 peach, 1 oz walnuts |
| **MEAL 4** | 6:00PM | 1 beyond meat burger patty, 1 GF bun, lettuce, tomatoes, red onion, 1 tbsp avocado oil mayo |
| Two 100-calorie snacks to be added when hungry. | | |

What about portion sizes? We don't need a food scale, but it does come in handy if we really want to focus on fitness goals, and if we have the time to measure our consumption. Here is a rough idea:

**Protein:** 4 oz meat (cooked), 2 eggs, 6 egg whites (or ¾ cup, measured raw), 1 cup cottage cheese or Greek yogurt, 1 cup beans or lentils, 1 scoop protein powder. Other vegan options for protein include hemp seeds, tofu, and seitan.

**Fats:** 1 tbsp all oils, 1 oz nuts, 1 oz nut butter, 1 oz seeds, 1/2 avocado, 6-8 small olives

**Carbohydrates:** 6 oz potatoes, sweet potatoes, yams, yucca (cooked weight), ¾ cup rice (cooked weight), ¼ cup quinoa (cooked weight), ¼ cup (dry) oatmeal (steel cut oats), ½ cup (dry) quick oats, 2 thick rice cakes - 6 thin square ones, 1 cup fruit, unlimited veggies,

**Condiments** - to be used in moderation - spices, herbs, sea salt and pepper, sugar-free salsa, tomato sauce, salad dressing, vinegars, mustard, ketchup, jam, maple syrup, Sriracha, soy sauce, Braggs.

**Some 100-calorie snack ideas:** 1 cup veggies with 1 tbsp dip, 1 small apple with 1/2 oz mixed nuts, 2 tbsp hummus with veggies, 10 corn tortilla chips, 1 slice whole grain toast with sugar-free jam, 2/3 oz dark chocolate, 1 cup shelled edamame, 1 small scoop frozen yogurt, 9 Kalamata olives, 2 cups air popped popcorn, 1 rice cake with 1 tsp nut butter, 2 tbsp guacamole w/celery sticks, 1/2 cup cottage cheese with 1/4 cup fruit, 1 oz goat cheese with cucumber slices, 1/2 cup Greek yogurt drizzle honey, 3 oz almonds and 1/2 cup applesauce with cinnamon, 20 baby corns dipped in soy sauce.

I know what you're thinking — what about **alcohol**? I am not a demon, you can still have some booze! We are human, and we are social creatures. So the occasional consumption of alcohol can be factored into your plan, but the key is moderation. If you know you are going to be consuming a few beverages — just lower your carb intake for the day (but not in excess, still have some carbs).

Remember that this is a lifestyle, not a diet! To break free from a dieting mentality, you have to get rid of those old false beliefs and create new ones. How can we ensure a sustainable nutrition plan?

**There are no REAL rules!** Eating should be customized to you and what works for your body and taste buds. Everyone is different.

**If it tastes good, makes you feel good, and supports your goals — eat it!** Learn to fuel your body from within and act from a place of love, not deprivation.

**Whole foods are always ideal for digestion, but they're not the be-all-end-all.** Try to nourish yourself from the inside, and your outside fitness goals will follow.

**If it has an end date, is a diet or a fad, and has a label attached to it, it is not sustainable.** Just don't do it!

**If it requires fancy pills, juices, shakes, coffees, or powders,** don't do it!

**If it makes you so hungry that you are angry, sick, or mean,** stop freakin' doing it!

**If it cuts out an entire food group, it is not sustainable in the long run.** Find your own unique nutritional balance that works for you.

That's it — that's my "eat for the rest of your life" or "try your damn best" nutrition plan in under 3,500 words! Focus on simple, high-quality, and long-term, and you will highlight the body you have and rock the shit out of it!

> *I tried every diet, from living on cabbage soup to fasting to Weight Watchers, and then came the frozen meals and the shakes. I realized that the more I took care of my body, eating what was good for me, then I felt happy and whole.*
>
> ~ ASHLEY GRAHAM

## ROCK WITH US

Write down a daily or weekly meal plan for yourself using my R.E.A.L tips. Then, take a screenshot and hashtag **#kissmycurvyassets** to show us the amazing plan you have, so that we can share in some of your ideas!

### DAY 1

MEAL 1 _____

MEAL 2 _____

MEAL 3 _____

MEAL 4 _____

SNACKS _____

### DAY 2

MEAL 1 _____

MEAL 2 _____

MEAL 3 _____

MEAL 4 _____

SNACKS _____

### DAY 3

MEAL 1 _____

MEAL 2 _____

MEAL 3 _____

MEAL 4 _____

SNACKS _____

# CHAPTER 14

# MOVE YOUR ASSETS ON YOUR OWN TERMS

*It's not so easy. I hate it just like anybody else. It's not fun. You do it because you want to feel good and it makes you feel good after you do it.*

~ JENNIFER LOPEZ

Just like nutrition, exercise plays only a small part in finally embracing, enhancing, highlighting and rocking the shit out of your body. By now, you must have guessed that I am not one for cookie-cutter anything, so there won't be workout regimens in this chapter. Instead, I will focus on how to fit exercise into your life on your own terms, without having it consume your every thought. Move your "assets" how *you* want to. Find ways to move your body that make you happy instead of feeling as though it's yet another chore on your daily list.

It's no wonder so many of us have a distorted relationship with food and with exercise! We are often taught that exercising or working out is a punishment for eating! "OMG, I better go heavy in spin class or go on a long forty-five minute run to make up for all the 'bad' food I've eaten this weekend." As a result, we feel terrible, guilty, and ashamed of our food choices.

Social media is packed with workout plan after workout plan. Models doing lunges and crunches, and telling you that to get a body like theirs, you have to buy their plans. But what if you don't even like working out? Or what if you don't want it to consume your life? Fitness is important, but it shouldn't overshadow everything else in our lives. Did you know that one hour of physical activity is only four percent of our day? Shouldn't that one hour be an hour when we can look forward to having some fun, while giving back to our bodies?

Exercise should be fun and rewarding, not a punishment or a death sentence for something we ate. We often think that exercise needs to be intense, or extreme, or high intensity, but in reality, *any* exercise is good for you! (Remember the 700 calories burned in a hot and steamy sex session!?) The key to sustaining any daily physical activity regimen is focusing on your *why*. Ask yourself why you exercise. Is it to punish yourself for eating those "bad" foods or to get rid of body parts you hate? Or do you exercise because you respect and love your body, and you want regain energy or relieve stress? Perhaps you are somewhere in the middle of these responses. Whatever your reason is, check in to see if it stems from a place of love and respect for your body. If it's not, I encourage you to shift your reasons. Find activities that make you feel good rather than bad. Find activities that let you play and have fun, rather than torture yourself. Learn to love exercise by respecting your body just as it is now. Focus on how being active makes you feel — emotionally, mentally, physically — and break free from associating food with exercise.

Wouldn't it be great to CHOOSE how you move your body? Let's think about activities we enjoy that might not involve living at the gym or in the Soul Cycle class. How about things like: tennis, yoga, squash, hip hop dancing, Pilates, hiking, dog walking, baseball, long runs, sprinting, stair climbing, ballet, belly dancing, Zumba, swimming, hockey, rock climbing, boot camps. The list is endless. Sure, lifting weights can increase your lean muscle mass, but these sports or activities can also yield amazing results, especially if you enjoy them!

So what do I recommend in terms of scheduling fitness into your weekly routine? Whatever works for you! Whatever works for your day-to-day lifestyle and schedule, and whatever is sustainable! I also recommend taking the approach of "Less is more!" As the old saying goes, "Too much of anything can be a bad thing," and that also includes too much exercise. Excessive exercise can actually cause health problems, especially if your diet is lacking in proper nutrition. More on this a little later.

Workouts are designed to stress the muscles, causing small tears that the body repairs; this then strengthens and builds muscle. The body needs time to adequately repair the tissue damage created by exercising. Vary your workout routine and allow for enough rest and recovery time to banish the boomerang weight-gain caused by overtraining and to keep your workouts from becoming boring for you and your muscles. The rest days are when the real magic happens in terms of getting you closer to your fitness goals.

But how do you know if you're overtraining? In order to prevent over-exercising, it helps to know what happens to the body when you're under too much physical stress. That way, you can recognize the warning signs.

Here are several signs of overtraining that'll indicate when you're pushing yourself a bit too far:

• Changes in your heart rate

• Trouble falling asleep and poor sleep quality

• Increased soreness

• Joint pain

• Moodiness, anxiety, or depression

• Fatigue or exhaustion

• Changes in your appetite

• Excessive thirst

• Digestive issues

• Irregular periods or changes to your menstrual cycle

But why do we have to worry about overtraining? Here's how it really kicks-you-in-the-ass, and not in a good way:

**Raises cortisol levels.** People battling weight gain are repeatedly told that they simply need to exercise more and cut calories, but in reality, this can damage your metabolism and can totally backfire. If you live in a caloric-deficit state because your exercise level is too high and food intake is too low, your body gets the message that it must slow down to save energy. You can wind up in a catabolic state that causes hunger, dehydration, and intense cravings for sugar or salt.

**Can lead to adrenal fatigue.** While moderation undoubtedly has positive effects on hormonal health, too much exercise without proper rest can cause chronic stress and lead to a severe type of adrenal fatigue. This is when the adrenal glands become so depleted that they stop producing enough of the crucial "stress hormones," including cortisol and types of adrenaline.

**Causes changes in mood and sleep.** Similar to adrenal fatigue, the glands that typically control the production of hormones responsible for keeping your mood perky can begin to malfunction when you over-exercise. Over-training can actually lead to depression and can also place the nervous system and the endocrine (hormone) system under undue stress. Additionally, it impacts sleep quality and can lead to insomnia. In very serious cases, overtraining has been connected with suicidal tendencies.

**Can negatively impact libido, menstrual cycles, and fertility.** Too much exercise can negatively impact the production of sex hormones (like testosterone and estrogen) associated with libido, fertility, and reproductive health. Some women stop getting consistent, or any, menstrual cycles. When your body gets the signal that it's being worked too hard, it causes your stress hormones to fire at a higher rate, which can lead to symptoms similar to premenstrual syndrome (PMS), including acne, insomnia, low libido, food cravings (think sugar addiction), and other hormone malfunctions. Side note - I didn't get my period for three years when I was in high school and excessively exercising, and I lost it more than a dozen times when I competed in fitness competitions. Knowing what I know now, I can't believe the internal damage I was causing myself!

**Leads to decreased strength and loss of muscle.** Rest! I just said it above! Your muscle tissues cannot rebuild themselves fast enough when you don't give them enough rest in between workouts.

**Raises inflammation and lowers immunity.** Overtraining can increase oxidative stress and damage, which leads to illness and faster aging.

Your immune system stops functioning properly when you're operating in "starvation mode," and you're more likely to become sick and heal more slowly. Overtraining is also associated with increased risks of infection, including respiratory tract infections.

**Can cause heart damage.** While moderate exercise is important for cardiovascular functioning, overdoing it is counter-productive. You might notice that overtraining can also result in an altered resting heart rate, since the body is working in overdrive in the same way that it does during an emergency.

**Screws with electrolyte levels.** Your muscles rely on fluids, magnesium, sodium, and potassium to stay healthy. Exercise can deplete you of all of these much-needed nutrients.

So, just like with our nutrition, we should exercise in moderation.

What do you like to do in terms of exercise? You might be a cardio junkie like I was about a decade ago. But when I decided to quit it with the excessive cardio and focus more on hitting the strength training, my body did amazing things. I was able to highlight my already amazing curves and assets by adding lean muscle. This doesn't mean I turned into Arnold Schwarzenegger. It means that everything was more toned, harder, leaner, smaller, and just had a better appearance. The biggest myth out there is the cardio myth — we need to stop our excessive relationship with cardio. When it comes to your body composition, doing too much cardio does not promote muscle growth and might actually break down existing muscle. So instead of spending long periods doing "traditional cardio," such as running on a treadmill, think about switching up your workout routine by kicking up the intensity and lowering the duration.

Here are some of the many benefits of such a change:

- Improved blood cholesterol levels

- Increased energy levels and mood

- Decreased blood pressure

- Increased oxygen used by muscles

- Increased insulin sensitivity (lower risk of diabetes)

- Increased resting metabolic rate (means body burns more calories all day)

- Reduced risk of stroke and heart disease

- Save that lean muscle, and continue to build it instead of letting the longer workouts burn it away!

When it comes to exercise and how it fits into your real life, let's use this awesome way to determine if it is good for YOU!

**What is your REAL exercise plan:**

| R | Right for your body type. We are all built differently. |
|---|---|
| E | Enjoyable and doesn't suck. |
| A | Adaptable when you are busy, travelling, or when life changes. |
| L | Lifelong. It should be something you can sustain forever and not short-term or extreme. |

Other than actually looking better and reaching your body goals through exercise, there are so many other benefits to moving your body:

**Better mood:** Within five minutes of exercising, you can feel happier! When you move those curves and assets, your brain releases serotonin, dopamine, and norepinephrine. These make you feel amazing! Boost your mood by moving that junk-in-the-trunk!

**Decreased stress:** You don't have to engage in intense exercise. In fact, low to moderate intensity exercise is better than high-intensity for stress reduction. Hatha yoga or a nice stroll to enjoy the sunshine can be amazing stress-busters.

**Mental strength:** Exercise that pushes you physically always helps you get tougher mentally. More mental toughness means better stress management. If you can handle a challenging spin class, just think of how you will be able to better take on your daily tasks in life — bring it on, world!

**Easy-peasy life:** If you can lunge and press twenty pounds or hike a mountain wearing a twenty pound vest, just think of how much easier your daily chores and tasks, like lugging groceries, gardening, or chasing the kids around with the soccer ball, will become. Wouldn't it feel so much better to take on those things with ease?

**Higher immunity:** When exercising, you sweat out toxins and bacteria. When your blood is pumping, you are also increasing the rate at which antibodies and white blood cells, which fight illness, run through the body. In addition, when you exercise, the release of stress-related hormones slows.

**Enhanced life:** When you move your body more, it just becomes easier to want to participate in this world. You feel better, you look better, and you move with ease. Life is short — make sure you move in it with ease!

**Graceful aging:** Exercise helps you maintain a healthy weight, which can help you age more gracefully. As we age, joints become stiffer, muscles shrink if they aren't used, and we have more aches and pains. But we can use exercise to ensure aging isn't such a process, and make it enjoyable and easy instead!

**Better zzz's:** Burn calories, burn energy, and when you hit the sack at night, you will be counting sheep deeper than ever!

**Energy explosion:** I wake up every day at 4 a.m.! I hit the gym for 4:45 a.m. sharp, like clockwork. I must say, this has helped me become so much more productive during the day, and I just get the most from my days from that morning burst of exercise endorphins. This doesn't mean you have to work out in the morning like me — an afternoon workout can re-energize you and take you out of the mid-day slump.

**Reduced anxiety and depression:** Exercise helps release those endorphins that keep us feeling good and keep our moods up. It is also actually proven to prevent depression and anxiety, and can be used as an aid for those struggling with those issues and needing to supplement their treatment.

To round out this chapter, I wanted talk about MUSIC TO MOTIVATE and help push your workouts or exercise to a new level. I compiled a list of *must-have* songs that are ALL ABOUT YOUR ASSETS — celebrating female curves and the female body, embracing your beauty, and rocking the shit out of what we have! Enjoy! **FIND THIS KICK-ASS LIST ON SPOTIFY – Under "Kiss My Curvy Assets," and rock away to it when you move your hot body!**

*Born This Way - Lady Gaga*
*Sexy Back - Justin Timberlake*
*Fat Boy - Max-A-Million*
*I'm Too Sexy - Right Said Fred*
*Bootylicious - Destiny's Child*

*Baby Got Back - Sir-mix-a-lot*
*All about the Bass - Meghan Trainor*
*Fat Bottom Girls - Queen*
*Low - Flo Rida*
*Booty - Jennifer Lopez and Iggy Azalea*
*Big Booty Bitch - Bombs Away*
*Anaconda - Nicki Minaj*
*Rump shaker - Wreckx-n-effect*
*Shake That Thang - Sean Paul*
*Milkshake - Kelis*
*Shake Ya Tailfeather - P. Diddy (featuring Nelly)*
*Shake That Ass - Eminem (featuring Nate Dogg)*
*My Humps - The Black Eyed Peas*
*Video - India Arie*
*Q.U.E.E.N - Janelle Monae and Erykah Badu*
*Big Girl (You are Beautiful) - MIKA*
*Work It - Missy Elliot*
*Hips Don't Lie - Shakira (featuring Wyclef Jean)*
*Unpretty - TLC*
*Scars to Your Beautiful - Alessia Cara*
*Most Girls - Hailee SteinfeldBiggie Smalls - CupcakKe*
*My Skin - Lizzo*
*Thunder Thighs - Miss Eaves*
*Shameless - Lissie*
*Sorry Not Sorry - Demi Lovato*
*Confident - Demi Lovato*
*Body Love Part 1 - Mary Lambert*
*Pretty Hurts - Beyonce*
*Whole Lotta Rosie - AC/DC*
*Big and Chunky - Moto Moto (featuring Will I am)*
*Fighter - Christina Aguilera*
*Firework - Katy Perry*
*F\*ckin Perfect - Pink*

# MOVE YOUR ASSETS...

*Girl on Fire - Alicia Keys*
*Raise Your Glass - Pink*
*Run the World (Girls) - Beyonce*
*Who Says - Selena Gomez*
*Just the Way You Are - Bruno Mars*
*What Makes You beautiful - One Direction*

There you have it! So many benefits of moving and shaking, other than just seeing the outer results! So how does moving your assets on your own terms help you embrace and rock the shit out of your body, and finally achieve those long-term fitness goals? Because it works for you! It is something you want to do. It is easier to implement something that's good for you when you also enjoy it. Try your best to fit in some form of strength training if you can, but otherwise, just find activities that you don't dread doing. For example, maybe twice a week, you can hit the local gym for a strength training workout, and then take two longer hikes with your partner, a dance class with your bestie, and a hot yoga class on Saturdays for date night. That is one amazing, fitness-filled week! Just like you need to empower yourself to love the skin you're in, you should empower yourself enough to know that you get to choose how you move your assets! And remember, exercise and nutrition are the smaller fish in the much bigger pond of rocking the shit out of your body!

*You've got to keep your body active, even if that means just turning on some music and dancing for an hour . . . That's how you'll prepare your bodies and your minds for greatness.*

~ MICHELLE OBAMA

## ROCK WITH US

Move your assets. Write out your plan to move your body for a week. Take a screenshot and hashtag **#kissmycurvyassets** so we can see you move **YOUR** body on **YOUR** terms!

MONDAY        _____

TUESDAY       _____

WEDNESDAY     _____

THURSDAY      _____

FRIDAY        _____

SATURDAY      _____

SUNDAY        _____

NOTES

_____

_____

_____

_____

_____

_____

_____

_____

_____

_____

_____

# CHAPTER 15

# CREATE SUSTAINABLE GOALS

*If you set out to do something and you give it your all and it doesn't work out, be willing to modify your goal slightly. Have the ability to look in another direction. A small shift could guide you to the real purposes in your life.*

~ HALLE BERRY

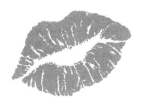

When I was younger, I was a "shoot for the moon" type of goal-setter. I would aim high and think, *What's the harm in thinking big?*" My mentality was always, "Go big or go home." I had to always be striving, always had to have a five-year plan, big dreams, and insane hopes, and I often set the bar so high that I ended up crashing and burning in the end.

Everywhere you look online, you see a "How to create goals" guide, like the S.M.A.R.T. goals strategy: "Specific, Measurable, Attainable, Realistic, Timely."[29] Let's keep this one simple, and break it down a little more:

**Specific:** A specific goal has a much greater chance of being accomplished than a general goal. To set a specific goal, you must answer the six "W" questions: *Who *What *Where *When *Which *Why.*

**Measurable:** Establish concrete criteria for measuring progress toward each goal you set. When you measure your progress, you stay on track, reach your target dates, and experience the exhilaration of achievement that spurs you on to the continued effort required to reach your goal.

**Attainable:** When you identify the goals that are most important to you, you begin to figure out ways you can make them come true. You develop the attitudes, abilities, skills, and financial capacity to reach them.

**Realistic:** To be realistic, a goal must represent an objective toward which you are both willing and able to work. A goal can be both challenging, yet realistic; you are the only one who can decide just how challenging your goal should be.

**Timely:** A goal should be grounded within a timeframe. If you want to lose two inches off your waist, *when* do you want to lose it by? But remember to set a realistic timeframe to achieve your goal.

# CREATE SUSTAINABLE GOALS

It's good to have both short-term and long-term goals. Short-term goals are defined as something you want to see happen in the next one to three month timeframe. They need to be aligned with your day-to-day life and take into account work, school, kids, spouse, and time commitments. They truly need to fit the S.M.A.R.T. principles listed above. In fitness, it's best to stop being so numbers-focused (i.e,. lose ten pounds pounds) and instead make it more about lifestyle changes.

More long-term goals can be defined as something you want to see happen in the next year. They still need to take into account your busy schedule and life, but these can dig deeper and be more grand. It never hurts to set higher long-term goals, and then smaller shorter term goals to help get you there!

So you have set your S.M.A.R.T. goals. Next you need to find a method of accountability. Support systems are key to help your keep your eye on the prize. Accountability is so important in goal-setting. Once you set intentions, sharing them with others who are supportive and will keep you accountable ensures follow-through. For some, this means a close friend; others choose to hire a coach or join a tribe or community of women with similar goals and lifestyles.

Regardless of which option you choose, you should also write down your goals. A vision board is another wicked way to view your goals every day and keep you accountable. I do up this easy-to-make bulletin board with clippings from travel magazines of places I want to go and green veggies to remind me to eat more green shit! I have pictures of dogs to remind me to get in nature with my dog more, and also some wicked photos of different body types to remind me that fitness comes in all shapes and sizes. It's in my office to keep reminding me daily of all of the little goals I am trying to achieve.

Finally, consistency will be key. in reaching those goals you are setting. Once you've set your goal, you need to come up with a plan that emphasizes consistent effort. The idea of goal-setting is to challenge yourself each time you set out to work toward your larger goal. Tracking progress will keep you more motivated and prevent you from getting sidetracked. Celebrate small changes and steps toward the bigger picture. Remember, you're not going to see changes all the time — you may also encounter plateaus. Be patient and gentle with yourself . . . Use journaling to track progress, be it in a planner, a little book, or even an app. Celebrate those small steps you are taking toward your fitness goals.

Let's talk some goals you can set that do not involve your body weight, your waist size, or your thigh thickness:

**Move your body more.** This could include taking more steps per day or using a tracker that sees how much you are moving! Make it your goal to move your body, and you will see those external goals without them being your sole focus.

**Take up a new sport, class, or hobby that involves moving your body.** This could be yoga, spin, soccer, anything really. Join a hockey team. Get a class pass at a local belly dance studio. Learning something new is always fun and exciting, so just try something that gets you moving.

**Complete a fitness challenge (something that isn't extreme).** Find things like the squat or push-up challenge, which take such little time and gives you little homework assignments every day.

**Meditate, or set daily affirmations**. The simple act of breathing more, or being still, can be goals that aren't just about the numbers and more about internal mental shifts.

**Set goals for a certain number of workouts per week.** Say you set your goal of four workouts per week — no matter how you choose to move your body, you are working toward a goal that's not focused on weight.

**Use more positive self-talk.** Look in the mirror and write down all of the things you are thankful for about your body. This is about losing the negative and gaining self-love, acceptance, or worth.

**Get better sleep.** Say you are stuck in the rat race of getting less than five hours of sleep per night. Setting a goal to get more sleep — closer to seven to eight hours — would be a great way to improve on your overall fitness goals. I talk about sleep a lot in this book because it is truly important on so many levels!

**Have more sex.** We know from the previous chapter how important orgasms are, as well as the calorie burn we get from sex, so this could be a great non-scale victory. Orgasm more often! That's a goal at the top of my list! I will say it one more time for the cheap seats in the back - HAVE MORE SEX!

**Eat more veggies.** More veggies mean better overall health. This is a wicked goal to push toward embracing and rocking that body!

**Get stronger.** Maybe set more personal best goals in the gym, for example, squatting heavier, doing more pushups, or just gaining more strength.

**Less dining out and take-out.** This one is about taking a not-so-healthy more processed lifestyle and creating more nourishing habits, for the end result of overall fitness!

**Eat breakfast.** Many of us skip breakfast and mistime our meals. Aim to eat every three hours to keep your metabolism working and to avoid being hangry (hungry and angry).

**Take the stairs more.** I remember going to Las Vegas and staying at the Wynn Hotel — there were sixty-three stories in that hotel. I was on the twenty-ninth floor. When we would return from shopping trips, lunches, and sightseeing, I would take the stairs up to my room, not the elevator. You better believe that even with the excessive drinking and calories consumed on that trip, I maintained my sleek physique because I was walking so much! Plus it just felt good to make my way up flight after flight — when I reached the top, it was such a great feeling.

**Be healthier for your children (or live longer).** Longevity is a great goal, as is having a better quality of life!

These are just a few great non-scale victories, but what things should we avoid or steer clear of and what things should we use to stay on track?

**Turn off the noise.** Screw society and social media. The fitness world focuses mainly on appearance and on this obsession with using exercise to obtain the "ideal." Fitspo, fitspiration, and hashtags are everywhere to derail us from being proud of our own fitness goals. We forget that we each have our own journey to take, our own ideals, and our own unique goals! Remember — fit bodies come in all shapes and sizes.

**Don't choose goals that hurt you.** Nix the fads, extremes, and harsh methods, and focus on sustainable long-term habits instead. As the saying goes, "*Slow and steady wins the race.*" There is no such thing as overnight success or healing, and if there is, it often comes at the cost of something quite important. Torture and scars are not methods that serve your overall long-term health and wellness.

**Focus on the feeling.** There are so many benefits to eating well, exercising, and setting health-based fitness goals that have nothing to do with ripped abs or a tight booty.

**Listen to your body — and head!** Does what you are doing to achieve your fitness goals feel good? The "no pain, no gain" method is an outdated one; when coaches or trainers preach that, I just want to tell them to fuck off! Respect your body's limitations and know that you don't have to be "beast mode" to see great results. One gym I went to had a puke bucket. A freakin' puke bucket of insanity! People used to find it funny when gym patrons worked so hard that they needed to throw up during a workout. Quite frankly, this baffled me and still pisses me off — throwing up means you aren't serving or benefitting your body. So to use this as positive reinforcement, when it is clearly abusing your body, is insane! It's okay to be a little out of breath during workouts, but to be pushing yourself to the point of puking, not a good idea!

**Kick diet culture to the curb.** If we keep seeing fitness as nothing more than a way to burn calories or punish ourselves for overindulging at dinner last night, it's always going to be a guilt-based obligation. Don't think of your workouts or your healthy meals in terms of what they're doing for your exterior body. Rather, focus on your interior experience of life. That way, the exterior will happen without dwelling on or obsessing about it.

**Don't eliminate food.** Remember that moderation, not starvation or deprivation, is your best companion. Stop the madness of "good" versus "bad" foods and instead focus on moderation and nourishing without obsessing. Do not fall into the diet trap of clean eating or forbidden foods. You can have your greens *and* your dessert (in fact, there are tons of yummy, wholesome, and nutritious dessert recipes out there. Yes, I just called dessert wholesome and nutritious!), and still benefit both your body and your mind. Remember that extreme restriction isn't healthy, mentally or physically. You and your body deserve to eat whatever the hell you want, and enjoy eating it, without so many rules.

So, there we have it. Setting S.M.A.R.T. goals, sustainable ones that are non-scale victories, will help you embrace your body and rock the shit out of your body while finding those long-term fitness goals!

*What I know for sure is this: The big secret in life is that there is no big secret. Whatever your goal for this year is, you can get there — as long as you're willing to be honest with yourself about the preparation and work involved. There are no back doors, no free rides. There's just you, this moment, and a choice.*

~ OPRAH

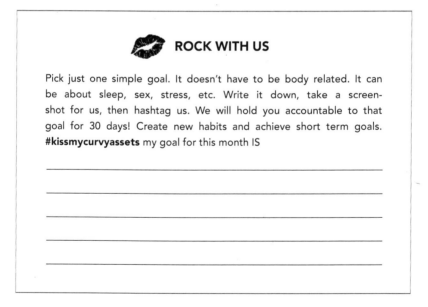

**ROCK WITH US**

Pick just one simple goal. It doesn't have to be body related. It can be about sleep, sex, stress, etc. Write it down, take a screenshot for us, then hashtag us. We will hold you accountable to that goal for 30 days! Create new habits and achieve short term goals. **#kissmycurvyassets** my goal for this month IS

_____

_____

_____

_____

_____

# CHAPTER 16

# CHECK YOUR H.A.T (HORMONES, ADRENALS, THYROID)

*I am in control of how I age, and I am in control of my health.*

~ SUZANNE SOMERS

You are busting your ass in the gym and laser-focused on nutrition — counting calories, measuring servings of food, and really focusing on your "plan." You are working your tail off, literally, but your body isn't changing. In fact, you are gaining weight instead of losing it. You look almost toxic. That tiny waist you once had now houses a spare tire around it — no matter the lengths you go to, you just cannot seem to see any progress. It's a losing battle. Everyone around you just rolls their eyes and scoffs when you emphasize how hard you are truly working at becoming healthy. They assume you are "cheating off plan" or "missing workouts."

But what they don't realize is there is a whole lot of shit going on internally that may be throwing your ultimate fitness goals for a total loop. Your endocrinological system might be out-of-whack, thus making it impossible to achieve those body ideals. I can tell you firsthand, when you have imbalanced hormones, it can lead you into a downward spiral that is tough to climb out of.

Don't worry, there are answers, there is help . . . but you have to check your H.A.T:

**H - Hormones**

**A - Adrenals**

**T - Thyroid**

First, let's break it all down, and then we'll talk about the M word and the P word (the secret fitness goal killers):

**M - Menopause**

**P - Perimenopause**

Hormones — everyone has 'em! They build bones, maintain muscle, and protect joints. They regulate breathing, fight stress, lower anxiety, relieve depression, and impact our sex drive and fertility. Whew! To say that they are important to the quality of your life is a huge understatement! When our hormones are balanced, they are awesome! But when they are out of balance, just watch out for the shit-storm they can cause! Hormones play a huge role in how we age, grow, and function, and any hormonal imbalances can cause diseases and major health problems.

Let's talk first about the three "minor" hormones, that really aren't minor at all! Estrogen, testosterone, and progesterone.

Estrogen is the most powerful hormone and is what makes a woman a woman. It's made up of three types of hormones — estrone, estradiol, and estriol. Elevated or even unusually low levels of estrogen can wreak havoc and have a significant impact on the quality of our lives.

**Symptoms of low estrogen:** weight gain - foggy thinking - bloating - bladder infections - itching - incontinence - sweating and hot flashes - allergies - depression - low sex drive (UGH!) - irritability - heart palpitations - weepiness - low bone density - trouble sleeping - painful intercourse

**Symptoms of elevated estrogen:** acne - anxiety and depression - polycystic ovarian syndrome (PCOS) - migraines - infertility - foggy thinking - ovarian cysts - red flush on face - mid-cycle period pain - gallbladder problems - puffiness and bloating - weepiness - rapid weight gain - mood swings - breast tenderness - heavy bleeding in periods

Sounds fun, right? On the other hand, an increase in estrogen can cause estrogen dominance, which can pave the way for cancer.

What about the other hormones such as testosterone? When in an optimal state, testosterone helps build strong bones and lean muscle. More importantly, it regulates our sex drive - holla!

**Symptoms of excess testosterone:** acne - unstable blood sugar - increased blood pressure - pain with ovulation - hair growth on face, chin, arms - infertility - deepened voice - ovarian cysts - polycystic ovarian syndrome (PCOS)

**Symptoms of low testosterone:** passivity - varicose veins - decreased interest in physical activity - increase fat on stomach and hips - weight gain - decreased mood and energy - lack of self-esteem/confidence - rounding of back, hunched shoulders - cellulite

Progesterone is supposed to be at its lowest in the first phase of your menstrual cycle. It increases ten days post-ovulation and decreases four days before your menstrual cycle begins. Progesterone is essential for pregnancy and the survival of a fetus, regulates blood sugar, supports sex drive, prevents PMS, protects against cysts on breasts, builds bones, is a natural diuretic, increases energy and stamina, protects against cancer, increases endurance, is a natural antidepressant, and helps thyroid function.

**Symptoms of low progesterone include:** painful, swollen breasts - miscarriage - anxiety and stress - weepiness - infertility - trouble sleeping - abdominal cramps - headaches - aggression - weight gain - heavy periods - swollen extremities - PMS - increased cancer risk - night sweats

So as you can see, these three "minor" hormones play a significant role in our lives. They impact our mood, as well as our physical, mental, and emotional health. If they are out of balance, we can really be thrown for a loop. Imbalances in these hormones all have some similar symptoms, so blood tests can help determine your hormone levels in order to assign a method of treatment: bio-identical hormones or natural remedies through nutrition, lifestyle, and bioavailable supplements.

The next crucial hormone regulator is our adrenal glands, which are located above our kidneys. When our adrenal glands are functioning optimally, our hormone levels are also balanced. However, when the adrenal glands are sluggish or low-functioning due to chronic stress and lifestyle factors, this results in what is known as adrenal fatigue or adrenal burn-out. Some factors that can cause adrenal fatigue include overwork, dietary imbalances, busyness, anemia, birth control pills, not enough rest, over-exercising or over-training, hormonal imbalances, inflammation, and infections.

**Symptoms of adrenal fatigue or burnout:** heart palpitations - inability to sleep - recurrent infections or illness - lack of calmness - achiness - more negative thinking and emotions - unstable blood sugar levels

A saliva test done by your physician or naturopath is a great way to test the adrenals; this usually measures your level of cortisol, which is our stress hormone.

**Symptoms of high cortisol levels include:** extra fat around neck - irritability - anxiety - excess hair growth - bloating - no sex drive - memory problems - skin problems, thin skin, bruising - irregular periods - weight gain - food cravings - lowered immune system - increased blood pressure - increased blood sugar - increased appetite

High cortisol levels, stemming from overtraining, not getting enough exercise, poor nutrition, and not getting enough sleep, can lead to insulin resistance. This can then lead to a yo-yo cycle of weight loss and weight gain, hence disrupting our fitness goals! You are not doing your body a favor by over-training and overexerting yourself physically when your adrenal glands are fried. If anything, further harm is being caused to your hormones.

We touched on the H and the A . . . now let's talk about the "T" word . . . Thyroid. The thyroid is a butterfly-shaped gland located in the lower part of our neck. It controls and regulates our metabolism and affects almost every system in our body. Stress can also affect our thyroid. If your thyroid isn't working right, you won't feel right. You don't want your thyroid operating too low or too high — you want it in the middle, just right (like Goldilocks and the three bears!). We can have either an underactive or an overactive thyroid. When we have an over-active thyroid (when there is too much thyroid production), it results in hyperthyroidism.

**Symptoms of hyperthyroidism include**: bulging eyeballs - getting upset easily - difficulty gaining weight - diarrhea - sometimes weight gain - nervousness - fatigue - warm, moist, coarse red skin - feeling agitated, wired, or unable to sleep - trembling hands

Conversely, when we have an underactive thyroid (when there is little to no thyroid production), it results in hypothyroidism. Hypo-thyroidism is typically most common after age forty; at least one in every five women in this age group suffer from this condition.

**Symptoms of hypothyroidism include**: weight gain - hoarse morn-ing voice - cold hands and feet - slow pulse rate - fatigue - high blood pressure - dry skin - slow thinking - constipation - little to no sex drive - difficulty losing weight - brittle nails - swelling - frequent colds and infections - depression - irrational and out-of-control be-havior - hallucinations - mental confusion - loss of memory

Something that has recently gained spotlight in the health and wellness industry is "Hashimoto's Thyroiditis," an autoimmune dis-ease that causes inflammation of the thyroid gland. Hashimoto's thyroiditis, named after Dr. Hakaru Hashimoto who discovered it in 1912, is said to have no cure and is often caused by hypothyroidism (too low levels of thyroid hormones). Those affected often see a lump in their throat of the front of their neck, have difficulty swal-lowing, or suffer from extreme fatigue. A blood test of your thyroid levels can often indicate whether any autoimmune disease is present. In recent years, I have seen such a huge influx of this condition, which inhibits a woman's ability to truly achieve their body goals.

Once you check your hormone levels, adrenal glands, and thyroid gland (H.A.T), you can rule out possible internal issues that might be keeping you from your fitness goals.

Now let's talk about the "M" and "P" words - menopause and perimenopause, the duo that are crushing fitness goals everywhere! I want to scream, cry, or hit something when I think about the number of women dealing with these conditions who think they are crazy or losing it!

Perimenopause is the time in a woman's life when physiological changes begin the transition to menopause. Menopause is the time when there have been no menstrual periods for twelve consecutive months. A woman can usually tell if she is experiencing symptoms of perimenopause because her menstrual periods start changing. I believe the REAL definition of perimenopause is "complete hormonal chaos about to throw the body and mind on a real path of disaster!"

Perimenopause typically begins several years before the natural onset of menopause. The timing of natural menopause varies, with the average age being fifty-one, but perimenopause may occur as early as age thirty-five for some. It feels like you're experiencing puberty again, with your hormones going for a complete chaotic journey — hot and cold flashes, crying for no reason, feeling alone, misunderstood, having unexplainable mood swings, and feeling as though you are living in an overall hormonal hellhole. I remember just feeling off. Not like myself. I knew something was wrong. When my family was always in hiding for fear of some emotional outburst I might throw at them, I knew something wasn't right.

Despite all my extreme efforts, I was having such a hard time losing weight and instead kept gaining weight in my mid-section. When I finally had the proper tests done by my naturopath, she sat me down and said, "You are imbalanced, bad! You are in perimenopause." I remember saying out loud, "My grandma and old women get menopause . . . I am only thirty-three!" *Why did no one tell me about this word, why did I think you had to be truly old to fall into this hormonal havoc and imbalance?*

| Suzanne Somers once defined perimenopause or menopause as the "Seven Dwarves (or moods) of Menopause": |
| --- |
| 1. Itchy 2. Bitchy 3. Sleepy 4. Sweaty 5. Bloated 6. Forgetful 7. All dried up . . . wow, sounds wonderful! |

As women, we need to talk more about women's health concerns; we need to increase awareness and let each other know that we are not alone in this suffering. We need to band together and find ways to treat these conditions holistically so that we can end this cycle of medicating ourselves as a band-aid solution.

Perimenopause and menopause have the same symptoms as imbalances in estrogen, testosterone, and progesterone (ETP), because that is what is happening in your body. You are not crazy; this is normal. However, you do not need to just live with it. There are holistic remedies to help manage your symptoms and help you thrive in your daily life.

Let's talk food! We can eat to nourish and balance our hormone levels. Here is a list of hormone-balancing foods that are easy to add to your nutrition plan:

| HORMONE BALANCING FOODS | Almonds (raw, unsalted) - Garlic - Apples - Meat - Avocado - Nuts - Beans - Olive Oil - Beets - Oranges - Blueberries - Pineapple - Broccoli - Shellfish - Cabbage - Sweet Potatoes - Eggs - Tomatoes - Flaxseeds - Wild Salmon |
| --- | --- |

Lowering consumption of sugars, and caffeine will help to balance your hormones, too. Replace coffee with teas (black, white, and green).

| HORMONE BALANCING SUPPLEMENTS | L-Carnitine (helps with the weight gain) - Boron (increases estrogen and testosterone) - Calcium with magnesium - Evening primrose oil - Fish oil (EFA - Omega 3s) - Vitamin D - Zinc (can be found in shellfish, beef, lamb, pumpkin, and sesame seeds) - Black cohosh, Chaste tree berry - Rhubarb - Saffron extract |
|---|---|

Other ways to balance hormones and ensure that adrenals are rested include:

• Get proper nutrition and ample calories (no fads or extreme diets!)

• Work out (but not in excess — keep it moderate)

• Add yoga and meditation

• Sleep (no gadgets before bed, ensure your bedroom is completely dark, no sleeping pills or wine before bed, go to bed by 9pm to ensure seven to eight hours of uninterrupted sleep)

• Magnesium epsom salt baths.

If the natural remedies aren't fully effective and you need additional support, you can consider Bio-identical Hormone Replacement Therapy (BHRT). This is where doctors or naturopaths help you discover hormone imbalances and create custom medications to balance them. This treatment is individually customized; your numbers need to be tested through frequent blood work to ensure proper dosage. For the thyroid, many doctors and naturopaths recommend desiccated thyroid, custom-made with t4 and t3, or some combination of the two, to get thyroid back to balance.

I cannot stress this enough: ladies, we need to talk about this frequently and be our own health advocates. A state of chaos, mind games, and unanswered suffering is not the way I want any woman to live. It is my mission to help women rock the shit out of their bodies and find their long-term fitness goals. Checking and balancing your hormone levels, adrenal glands, and thyroid (H.A.T) will help you to get there. If something seems off, listen to your body — your intuition is always right.

*I see menopause as the start of the next fabulous phase of life as a woman. Now is a time to "tune in" to our bodies and embrace this new chapter. If anything, I feel more myself and love my body more now, at 58 years old, than ever before.*

~ KIM CATTRALL

---

 **ROCK WITH US**

Take a pic of yourself holding your blood work results for hormones and thyroid from your doctor or naturopath. **DO IT**! Then hashtag **#kissmycurvyassets** to show you are taking your internal health into your own hands.

---

## NOTES

_____

_____

_____

_____

_____

_____

# CHAPTER 17

# WASH YOUR MOUTH OUT WITH SOAP - STOP WITH THE SWEAR WORDS

*Nobody is perfect. I just don't believe in perfection. But I do believe in saying - this is who I am and look at me not being perfect! I'm proud of that.*

~ KATE WINSLET

When we were kids and we used foul language, our parents would threaten us with the ever famous line: "I'm going to wash your mouth out with soap!" I can actually say that this did happen to me, and it didn't taste good — it also did not stop me from swearing (as you will notice from the many cuss words throughout this book)!

As adults, a great chunk of our vocabulary continues to be laced with swear words, but I'm not talking about the usual F bombs. These swear words, when spoken constantly and even mindlessly, have the power to shape our sense of self-worth and impact our self-esteem, which reprograms our mental and emotional mindset into a negative one. Let's examine some of these "swear" words a little more deeply and see how we can replace them for ones that promote a body positive mindset.

Let's start with the big one - the F word - Failure.

**Failure** means:

1. An act or instance of failing or proving unsuccessful; lack of success

2. Non-performance of something due, required, or expected

3. A subnormal quantity or quality; an insufficiency

4. Deterioration or decay, especially of vigor, strength, etc.

5. A person or thing that proves unsuccessful[30]

Some say that failure is a necessary precursor to ultimate success, yet we view failure as this negative and terrible thing. Just look at the life stories of Oprah, Thomas Edison, and major sports stars — they fall down over and over again, only to rise up and skyrocket into greatness. Failure is a part of life; messing up, stumbling along the way on our (*insert the type of journey you're on*) is what shapes us into who we are and ensures our successes. We actually benefit from failing. It's easy to see why we fear failures, screw-ups, and unknowns when you consider how they are perceived, but if we realize their value, we can move forward with a more positive mindset. What if we reframed our definition of failure? What if we viewed it as part of the process on our path to success? What if we found perseverance and opportunity as a result of our stumbling blocks? I know what you're thinking: "But Lori, failing sucks ass!"

Failures, screw-ups, and unknowns help us build our characters. Let's talk about some things we can do to respond when we "fail" or hit those speed bumps:

**Acknowledge the emotions you feel.** There is a reason they are surfacing. Reflect on them.

**Process those feelings and emotions.** Sit with them for a while and don't disregard them. Reflecting and processing helps you learn from your mistakes and keeps you pushing forward to success.

**Stop the blame game.** It's no one's "fault" — sometimes things or events happen that are outside of our control.

**Acknowledge any slip-ups and refocus on the steps you can take to correct them.** You are bound to keep repeating the same mistakes if you don't take time to find out why they occurred.

**Take action** to keep pushing ahead.

**Don't give up.** Setbacks often make us want to throw in the towel or curl up in a ball in the corner. We are all human, we all have detours in life — the key is to keep your eye on the prize and carry on putting one foot in front of the other. Recognize that these little mess-ups are normal and often necessary to find success.

Let's talk about the next big swear word - the S word - Starvation.

**Starvation** means:

1. To die or perish from lack of food or nourishment.

2. To be in the process of perishing or suffering severely from hunger.

3. To suffer from extreme poverty and need.

4. To suffer for a cause or lack of something needed or craved. Starvation is an extreme form of malnutrition.[31]

If our body doesn't get the nutrients it needs, it won't be able to maintain itself, grow properly, and fight off disease. If we don't eat, our body will deteriorate. First, our mental and physical performance will start to suffer. Eventually, our body's systems begin to shut down to conserve energy. Often, crash diets that promise quick results are masked by fancy packaging but are ridden with starvation-style weight loss techniques.

What happens when we starve the body? In the beginning, the answer depends on how much we currently weigh, whether we eat insufficient food or nothing at all, our age, our medical condition, and many other factors. Generally, during the beginning stages of starvation, we will experience fatigue, dizziness, dry or scaly skin, and weakness, as well as intense hunger. Our body is responding to the lack of food, which it needs for energy, by firing signals to our brain to do something about it. Starvation causes a decrease in cognitive function. Like every other part of our body, the brain needs nutrients and energy to function optimally.

Our mood will likely change as we become preoccupied by thoughts of food. We might feel anxious, irritable, angry, withdrawn, and depressed. As we continue on this path of destruction, we might start experiencing gastrointestinal disturbances, lower body temperatures, hypersensitivity to noise, water retention, and decreased libido. Our immune system won't be able to produce antibodies to fight infections, meaning we will get sick more often. Our metabolism decreases as our body tries to conserve as much energy as possible. Weight loss occurs as our body depletes fat stores, but the body's main focus is on burning lean muscle.

Eventually, failure to get sufficient nutrients will lead to permanent damage. We'll experience tooth decay and a weakening of our bones due to insufficient calcium. We'll experience hair loss due to a lack of protein and nutrients. Our organs will begin to shut down due to the lack of energy and nutrients. Our heart muscles will weaken, resulting in complete system failure or death. All of this in the quest to be size __. Lord help us — this all sounds serious, and it is. Think about the damage you are doing to your body to be some size you aren't supposed to be!

Many of us get roped into the latest and greatest fad, thinking that we have to be hungry or suffer to see results, but in reality, the damage being done is far more than we realize we had signed up for. I remember reading this quote by Kate Moss when I was younger: "*Nothing tastes as good as skinny feels.*"

What?! Actually, pizza tastes better than being skinny feels. Chocolate tastes better than skinny feels, and wine does, too! Being properly nourished with actual food tastes better than being skinny feels. What does this tell young girls when they read such a statement? Do we need to go into beast mode and suck up what we feel when we are in this state of starvation, since being skinny is way more important that fueling ourselves with the proper nutrients to live a thriving life? We need to lose this swear word, as well as abolish the concept of ever allowing ourselves to get stuck in the rat race of starvation diets.

In addition to the words "failure" and "starvation," "perfection" (this word simply irks me!) is another word that skews us emotionally and mentally on our quest to self-acceptance.

**Perfection** means:

1. The state or quality of being or becoming perfect.

2. The highest degree of proficiency, skill, or excellence, as in some art.

3. A perfect embodiment or example of something.[32]

Society has created such a ridiculous idea of perfection that all of us try to live up to every single day. We feel like we have to look and act a certain way. We're compelled to exercise and change the way we were built in order to fit into some mold. We scroll through those Instagram feeds, seeing the highlight reels of everyone's "perfect" bodies and lives. But why do we equate having the perfect booty with having the perfect life? Why should our external body or appearance dictate or define who we truly are?

No one is perfect, yet everyone strives for perfection everywhere they go. Have you ever sat back and actually thought about all of your flaws? Of course you have from time to time; we all do. But have you taken the time to consider how your flaws are actually what define you and make you the amazing being you are? "I came across the term "flawsome" in a meme, and I just loved the concept. "Flawsome" means someone who embraces their "flaws" and knows that they are awesome regardless. I FREAKIN' LOVE IT!

Truth be told, I don't think that I would have any idea who I am without my flaws. There is so much beauty in our imperfections — they set us apart from everyone else. The world would be a very boring place if we all fit the same mold, with the same look, the same size, and the same personality traits. *Stepford Wives,* anyone? I choose to be perfectly imperfect and embrace all of me. The word "perfection" has a negative connotation and energy associated with it, so we either need to reframe our perception of perfection or abolish that word from our vocabulary. Be perfectly imperfect and love yourself, because being comfortable in your own skin is the most beautiful thing of all. To me, *that* is the epitome of perfection — loving and embracing everything that makes me who I am.

Another word that gets thrown around in the diet industry is "deprivation."

**Deprivation** means:

1. To remove or withhold something from the enjoyment or possession of (a person or persons)

2. Going to extreme lengths in action, habit, opinion, etc.,

3. Exceeding what is usual or reasonable; otherwise known as immoderate or extreme behaviour,

4. Very strict, rigid, or severe; drastic; an extreme measure.[33]

The word just sounds nasty when it is defined. Why do we want to deprive ourselves or put ourselves in a state of extreme deprivation to achieve our fitness goals? What if we reframed our perspective and replaced it with the word "nourish" instead? Wouldn't that provide a more enjoyable life, along with more sustainable fitness goals?

Instead of punishing our bodies with deprivation to achieve our body ideals, why not embrace what we have and work toward our goals using nourishment as our go-to tool? We could replace the concept of deprivation with "moderation," thus getting rid of the "all-or-nothing" mentality and the need to be restrictive or eliminate anything altogether. Food deprivation, or restrictive eating, may cause us to dislike healthy nutritious foods. What happens when we are told we cannot have something? Those "forbidden" or restricted foods end up triggering us to binge or overeat. When we use deprivation as a weight loss tactic or a way to get our fitness goals back on track, it is a short-term, band-aid solution and will lead to a harmful long-term, yo-yo dieting game. We will only sustain our fitness goals in the long run and wholeheartedly learn to embrace our bodies when we a) use moderation as a technique and replace the word "deprivation" with "nourishment," b) have knowledge of the vast variety of nutrient-dense foods available to us, and c) realize we don't have to go "without" and can enjoy everything in moderation.

Engulfed in all these health and fitness trends, diet jargon, and diet plans is another buzz word, perhaps even more subliminally dangerous than the ones previously mentioned: "Transformation."

**Transformation** means:

1. The act or process of transforming

2. The state of being transformed

3. Change in form, appearance, nature, or character.[34]

I don't know about you, but I am happy being myself. Sure, I want to tweak a few things, sculpt or highlight a few areas, maybe lose a few inches . . . but why would I want to transform into someone else? I am me, and I am pretty darn awesome just the way I am. Celebrate yourself, your body, your efforts. Highlight your areas, but don't transform anything. Don't change! Focus on yourself and be the best version of yourself you can be. There is no need to turn into someone else. The whole idea of these transformations or empty promises that most new programs claim is to bring in the comparison game. They show these before-and-after pictures, and we then compare ourselves to their journey, our hopes all high, thinking that we, too, will completely change. However, we need to remember that we are our own beings and our bodies are unique. Replace "transform" with "highlight" or "accentuate" to appreciate and love what you already have.

When I was working on this chapter, there were so many words that truly hit me in terms of their negativity about body image. Words that got my back up against a wall and had me just feeling blah or pissed off when I heard them. We should never have to feel that way our their daily lives. If words have the power to make or break someone's mood, imagine how your mind, body, and soul feel when you are constantly using words with negative connotations. Constantly repeating words such as failure, deprivation, starvation, perfection, heck, even the word "diet," can do a number on us, mentally as well as on a cellular level when trying to heal our hormones and any other health conditions. If our body listens to our thoughts, imagine how much power our vocabulary can wield over our lives.

The word **"diet"** embodies all the four words we discussed in this chapter. How?

Think about it: In hopes of attaining some fitness or body goals, we jump into a new regimen with comparison as our master, chasing unrealistic illusions of what it means to be beautiful, fit, and socially acceptable (perfection). We partake in said diet (extreme or fad), restrict ourselves from eating certain foods (deprivation), and even go to extremes — we end up skipping a meal or two, or perhaps stop eating for a few days altogether, or even develop a detrimental health condition from constant lack of nutrient rich food (starvation). This vicious cycle continues for some of us until we become sick of feeling like we are not enough or sick of not being our true selves; however, some of us won't wisen up until something drastic takes place in our lives, such as a health diagnosis, or even the brink of death itself. Stop it, just freaking stop the madness!

Let's equate our relationship with food as a way of recharging our physical and mental battery or gas tank. You wouldn't be able to use your cellphone if it was constantly at a really low battery level, nor would you be able to drive your car on an almost empty tank for too long. Sooner or later, you would need to refuel or recharge. Similarly, the food we eat on a day-to-day basis is fuel for our body. There is no one-size-fits-all, cookie-cutter meal plan; we each have unique biological makeups and hence need our own special blend of bioavailable nutrients. We need to reframe our mentality from "diet" — aka "die"-t — to one in which we fuel and nourish our bodies with a variety of foods that make us feel good.

Stop saying those swear words, or I'm going to wash your mouth out with soap. I mean it! Remember that any struggle and stumbling block you encounter pushes you one step closer to success. Don't give up on yourself. Nourish your body, fuel it, and be kind to it with ample calories. Keep it all — everything in moderation, nothing is off limits. Be flawsome! Embrace your flaws, because they are what make you you! Rock what you've got! It is empowering to be ourselves and just highlight or accentuate what makes us truly amazing, unique beings! Eliminate this foul and negative language toward yourself and embrace your curves and assets. Celebrate them and and forge ahead to those sustainable, long-term fitness goals!

> *It's important to keep a balanced diet, but I'm not a fan of deprivation. If I want a cheeseburger, I'm not only going to have the cheeseburger, but I'm going to enjoy that cheeseburger.*
>
> ~ HEIDI KLUM

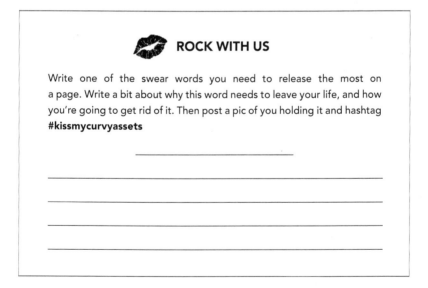

### ROCK WITH US

Write one of the swear words you need to release the most on a page. Write a bit about why this word needs to leave your life, and how you're going to get rid of it. Then post a pic of you holding it and hashtag **#kissmycurvyassets**

_____

_____

_____

_____

_____

# CHAPTER 18

# PAVE THE WAY TO BETTER BODY IMAGE FOR FUTURE WOMEN

*I'm never going to starve myself for a part. I don't want little girls to be like "Oh I want to look like Katniss, so I'm going to skip dinner."*

~ JENNIFER LAWRENCE
(ON HER ROLE IN THE HUNGER GAMES)

Growing up, I was like a sponge. If someone commented about their weight, I would internalize it and associate it with myself. Remember my story - I was actually called "chunky bum" by my family. Try bringing that with you through your childhood and teenage years without needing help from Dr. Phil. I was never a big kid, but I grew into my body at a young age. I mentioned before that kids actually called me "thunder thighs" on the playground (in hindsight, when looking back at old pictures, I actually didn't have big legs at all, so those comments were more about those saying them and less about me). In my teenage years, I never felt at home in my own skin. I was always trying to run with the crowd, fit in, look the same as everyone else. Back then, you never wanted to stand out or be unique. I wish someone would have taken me aside and said, "You are an amazing being just the way you are. Quit trying to be like everyone else, that's boring." I wish someone would have told me when I embarked on my quest for fitness and the "perfect" body that perfect doesn't exist and you need to create your own damn body ideals and ignore anything pushed upon you.

When I started writing this book and working on this movement, I had my daughter in mind, and my future granddaughter. I would give anything to have them not feel the pain, the self-abuse, the body-shaming I put myself through for over three decades. I want this movement to help millions of women everywhere change their mindsets, reprogram their way of thinking, and finally embrace and rock the shit out of what they have been blessed with. This in turn will filter on to the future of the female population. Just think if you could go back two or three decades and know what you know now. My life would have been quite different — my mindset, my self-esteem, even the direction of my life might have changed with more body confidence. I couldn't be saved from the madness I endured for so long, but I can help stop this madness from trickling down for future generations of women.

Little eyes are always watching. You might have a daughter,

niece, or some other little being who watches your every move. If you are dieting, they are absorbing what you are doing. If you are putting on clothing and commenting on how "fat" or "thick" you are, they are little sponges taking in and mimicking all that you say or do.

For years, I was a fitness competitor, and I was very conscious of never saying the word "diet" and always trying to keep a positive body image around my daughter and son for fear they would internalize it. One day, my then-four-year-old son walked into the washroom and stood on the scale and said, "I hate this thing, it never gives a good number, it's stupid." He must have seen me week after week, day after day, defining my self-worth by some number. He picked up on the pain it caused. Fast forward almost five years later, to when he was 10 (just a few years ago). He came into the room where I was sitting and said, "Mom, where is that metal thing that used to be on the floor in the washroom?" I had put it away in a closet, never to be seen again. I responded, "You mean the scale?" Yes, that was it. He replied to me, "I want it 'cause I need to lose some weight and it will give me a number. Online it says I should be X pounds, so then I will know how much I have to lose." I was mortified. Not only had he internalized some bad habits he learned from me, but he combined them with some nonsense he watched on a Youtube video about the ideal body weight for a ten-year-old boy. Goodness!

I have a client who has three daughters. Her loathing of her body for a decade has now created a whole slew of body image issues for her now-teenage daughters. You see, they saw their mother complain about her fat thighs and her mom belly. They saw her hating her body, and knew that they were a product of her. They now see their legs as fat, feel dread at ever being moms for fear of getting a mom stomach, and engage in self-abuse of their own bodies. Dieting was a staple in my client's household, so now any time these young girls are feeling badly about themselves, they punish themselves with deprivation and starvation. "I gained a pound, and in turn, I learned I need to not eat to punish myself for it." Little eyes are always watching. Even when you don't think they are.

We may try our best to keep our negative body image inside, but it shows on our faces, in our eyes, and in how we carry ourselves. As we start to focus on ourselves and our body image and embrace those curves and assets, how do we ensure our daughters (and sons) have a more positive body image than we did? Here are some ways we can help them set the stage for self-love, body-positive thinking, and owning their own shit in the future:

**Pay attention to how you talk about your own body.** Are you calling yourself fat? Are you constantly looking in the mirror and complaining about how you need to lose five pounds? Think about how you act when you need to find an outfit for an event. Are they seeing you try on all your clothing, only to throw it aside and say that you hate how it fits or how you look in it? *You* are the most important role model your children have. Not Britney Spears, not *Dora the Explorer,* YOU!

I remember my daughter coming to me once and telling me that she would never have skinny legs, that her legs would always be fat. My response to her was simple. "Well, I don't have skinny legs, I have strong legs, I can lift so many heavy weights. I don't aspire to have skinny legs, I want strong and shapely legs." She looked at my legs and agreed that she also liked the strong look. I also showed her tons of pictures of my clients, all very strong, curvy, and with different shapes and sizes of legs. I told her that all of them had the most amazing legs — *their* legs. No one was the same, but they were all amazing. To this day, even at sixteen-years-old, she aspires to just be strong. The word skinny doesn't exist in her vocabulary anymore. I try to talk about my body in a positive light as much as I can. "Wow, I love how my butt looks in these jeans - POW POW!" I try to talk about food in a positive light. "That salad was amazing, loaded with tons of healthy fats and just so many nourishing nutrients." If you keep a positive mindset about moving your body, nourishing your body, and seeing your body — these young girls will follow suit.

**Have an open dialogue with the younger generation.** Ask them how they feel about images on social media or how they feel about their bodies. Keep the dialogue open to be able to talk about what makes them tick in terms of their own body image. Educate them on self-love, self-acceptance, self-worth. Help them use tools like the three Ms: meditation, mantras, and motivation.

**Help them to pick activities they love and to move their bodies.** Physical fitness means far more than just reshaping our booties and finding a six-pack. It feeds our souls to move our bodies. Help young girls to find what they are passionate about. For example, my daughter hates the gym. You would think she would love it, being part of my gene pool, but she doesn't enjoy it. So she walks the dog; sometimes she goes to the gym, but instead of strength training, she enjoys playing on her phone as she rides the bike. I don't care what she does, as long as she moves her body for overall health and wellness. Encourage a healthy dialogue about physical strength and the importance of maintaining a healthy lifestyle when speaking with the younger generation.

**Let them cook with you and find a variety of nourishing foods they enjoy.** The more you expand their palettes to all the foods out there, the more your children will want to fuel themselves with it. Kids love to help! They love being little chefs, and they love eating their own creations. My favorite is the salad bar. Put out tons of selection and variety, then let your kids pick what they want. My son loves to cook with me, and while we are cooking, I educate him on what the foods are doing for his body.

**Use the term "Fitness comes in all shapes and sizes" as much as you can.** I try to have magazines, books, and images on my computer that are as diverse as possible in terms of body shapes. Many young girls develop eating disorders, starting with the magazines that show ultra-thin models, rather than a variety of ideals and norms.

**Don't comment on the size or shape of your daughters' or young girls' body parts.** This will lead to nothing but self-consciousness and fluctuating self-esteem. I am very careful of this when I compliment younger girls. For example, if they have a beautiful dress on and they look super cute, I make it more about them and less about the dress. "Wow, your eyes really glow bright in that dress!" The *girls* are the beautiful beings, not the piece of fabric they are wearing. Or "Wow, the green in that dress really makes your green eyes stand out — so stunning!" Less about body, and more about other traits standing out. I once saw a little girl in the most sparkly dress — she was the belle of the ball. When I praised her, I was conscious to point this out. "Wow, you almost floated in here, you just look so happy and are beaming with light right now." I made it about how she was such a stand out, and less about the fancy dress she was wearing.

**Let them know they're more than just their bodies.** In our appearance-obsessed culture, we need daily reminders that we're more than how we look. As women, we've become fixated on making ourselves look good, but what about all of the other things that make us well . . . us? We've each got strengths, talents, quirks, and flaws that make us unique. Teach your daughter and other young women that they are more than their bodies — they are heart, soul, spirit, passions, dreams, hopes, knowledge. Show them how to feel empowered by who they are and to truly understand that the way they look is secondary. Embrace those flaws, own their bodies, and to not let anyone create their ideals for them. They choose who they want to be, and they highlight what God gave them in their amazing bodies!

**Be open about discussing sex and sexuality.** I can't stress enough the importance of sex not being such a taboo topic. Why can't we talk about orgasms with our kids? Why can't we talk about masturbating, sex, love in relationships? Open communication is so important. Rape, sexual assault, and bullying are all topics we have a hard time discussing openly with our kids, yet we are petrified that it could happen to our little ones. So why not get the vocabulary going about it all early? Lesbian, gay, transgender — why are we waiting until they are in high school to educate them and help them learn that the world is a very diverse place, that it's okay to be different, that it's okay to talk about sex and sexuality openly without the fear of being judged. Where I live, the local education system ensures that sex education is a part of the curriculum from the primary years and touches on many of these topics. But I can remember when it was time for my daughter to take the workshop, she was mortified. She was six. I was driving her to school, and I openly talked about all that she was about to learn. But she had this fear that others would judge her for knowing stuff, for being educated. I always try to lighten the subject and inject some comedy whenever I can. As we were walking into the school, I yelled out at the top of my lungs, "Who is ready to learn about penises and vaginas today?" My daughter was mortified and tried to ignore me, hoping no one knew she was with me. My two-year-old son was in the stroller, and he yelled back with both hands in the air, "MEEEEE. Me mamma - penis!" as he pointed to his. Parents looked at me with embarrassment, and all I could think was, *We all* *have penises or vaginas, why aren't we talking about them?* When I was growing up, I remember we didn't talk about periods. At all. It was this off-limits topic. We called it stupid things like, "Aunt flow just came to town!" Jesus! God forbid if anyone ever knew you had your period. GASP! I remember my best friend, Terri-Lynn, and I were in our seventh grade music class — of course, it will be labelled the "white pants story" for decades to come. She stood up to get her homework back and there it was — staring right at the class — the white pants, with the massive bloody period stain on the back of them. She was mortified. I gave her my sweater to wrap around her waist, and she headed home shortly after. The sad part in all this was that she hid out for a month and missed school until everyone forgot about it, because she felt like she had no other option. The same thing happened to another friend, Jodi, about a year later. And I remember the boys starting to tease her, and bringing up the "white pants story" to my other friend. My response was a very loud and bitter, "We have vaginas, this means we will have periods, we will bleed, we will need this to have all your freaking babies one day! Be happy you don't have to worry about tampons, pads, or childbirth, and leave us the heck alone!" They didn't bother us girls about it again. Another such instance took place when I asked the teacher in my high school English class if I could be excused to go to the washroom. You see, my teacher, an older male, who I believe secretly hated me, said no. I had no problem holding my tampon up high in the air at the front of the class and explaining very loudly that I had my period and needed to change my tampon at that exact moment. He turned to-mato red, and let's just say that he never questioned my bathroom habits again. Why do we let sex and human nature stuff become so taboo and embarrassing? Talk about it young, and it won't be such a crazy or off-limits topic.

If we don't walk the walk and talk the talk ourselves, then we can't pave the way for the future generation of kick-ass, empowered females. The bottom line is that if we are full of shit and still dislike our bodies, are still on this impossible quest to fit some insane ideals, are still talking negatively to ourselves about our own body, are not embracing our own shit — then how are we to expect future women to do these things? If we speak up, stand out, or make a change in the norms laid out for us, future women won't have to struggle like we did. If we rock the shit we have and embrace our own bodies, we can then help other young ladies gain that same self-acceptance!

*One thing my mother did is that she never looked in the mirror and said "I'm so fat," or "I'm so ugly I need to go on a diet." Projecting that onto yourself is only going to make your daughter or son think that of themselves. Because they are a product of you.*

~ ASHLEY GRAHAM

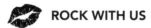 **ROCK WITH US**

Share a pic with your kids or someone from a younger generation making a healthy meal or exercising: show us how you're helping the next generation feel better about their bodies and their fitness. Hashtag **#kissmycurvyassets**

## NOTES

# CHAPTER 19

# EMBRACE YOUR CURVES AND ASSETS

*God made a very obvious choice when he made me voluptuous; why would I go against what he decided for me? My limbs work, so I'm not going to complain about the way my body is shaped.*

~ DREW BARRYMORE

Be body-positive. Accept your body. Just love yourself. Easy, right!? We have been using all these chapters to find ways to self-love, self-acceptance, confidence, and esteem. We have methods to the madness. But how does all of this really come into play? After years of abuse, self-bullying, and not accepting ourselves, how do we truly learn to embrace our curves and assets? How do we learn to accept and highlight all of our "curves" and "edges", or how bout those "perfect imperfections" - thanks, John Legend![35] Let's get ready to start embracing ourselves. It's so much less tiring to actually be empowered to accept and own every curvy, shape, edge, or jiggle.

**Admire yourself like you would admire your best friend. Own that goddess power within you.** We see our best friends as the goddesses that they are, yet are so hard on ourselves. How would you treat your best friend? Try treating yourself with a little more of that kindness.

**Compliment yourself often.** When you put on those jeans, tell yourself how rockin' your ass looks! If you have a good hair day, say it out loud to yourself. Watch your inner confidence soar!

**Make lists of all of the things you love about your body.** Do this often. Find a quiet space and type or write down in a journal all of the amazing parts of your body.

**When the negative talk comes out, replace it with something positive.** Challenge yourself to come up with something positive every time you have a negative thought. The positives outweigh the negatives.

**Quiet your inner critical voice.** And when it creeps back up, focus on your breath and don't allow your inner Negative Nelly to ruin the party. "Shut up, Susan!"

**Have a body positive mentor**. Find someone you look up to who embodies the movement, and surround yourself with their energy and flow.

**Actually sit and eat your food and enjoy it.** Stop thinking about calories, or macros, or good vs bad and enjoy every bite, every chew, every taste.

**When you move your body, be grateful you can.** Some are not so lucky.

**Do a photoshoot.** One of those boudoir shoots where you can put on a sexy outfit - or rock it in the flesh. A picture is worth a thousand words, and it's amazing how much of a sex goddess you will actually find in yourself when you see those hot pics!

**Take a pole dancing or burlesque dance class.** This can feel like the most fun and liberating thing you've done, and you can see yourself for the sexy being you are. I went with my best friend Patti once, and we actually died laughing at each other and had the greatest time of our lives. We realized that we were not sexy like the instructor, but we embraced our hotness and tried our best . . . and had an insane belly laugh while we were at it. It felt good to be silly and just let loose.

**Highlight your flaws.** Forget about just accepting your flaws — why not accentuate them? For example, a big round ass often looks better when you wear tight clothing to show off the curves instead of trying to hide them under baggy clothing.

**Remember *why* your body is what it is.** Are you a mom? Did you birth an amazing child to get those stretch marks on your belly? Are you sixty-five-years-old and wiser about the important things, ready to accept the curves and assets you have been blessed, the wrinkles, the looser skin?

**If you don't like it, change it.** I've talked a lot about accepting your body just as it is. But if you really do want your legs to be smaller, hit some spin classes and rock out some shaping and sculpting leg workouts. If you have loose skin on your tummy and you truly can't embrace and accept, change it. I'm not saying surgery is the answer, but it exists for a reason. If it is something that truly is hard for you to embrace, change it. You control your body, and you have the power to change things and be okay with it.

**Get social.** It's easy to loathe your body and never want to leave the jogging pants and baggy t-shirt. But it is so empowering to get yourself all dolled up and head out for a night on the town with girlfriends. Wine, appies, taking in a show, and just socializing to learn to embrace your body. You may dread doing it, but I promise you that once you are out and putting yourself in that social atmosphere, it will empower you to feel better about yourself.

**Read a good book.** There are so many amazing and inspiring books out there to not only feed your soul but to make you thankful for the body you have. They can range from books about self-help, self-longing, and women's issues, or to a good biography in which a woman overcomes tragedy and rocks this world. I love a good book that lifts me up, and shows me that I am pretty darn lucky to have what I have in my life and body.

**Clean out your closets — not the skeletons in your closet, your actual closet.** Why are we holding onto the jeans from ten years ago that are two sizes too small and haunt us on an almost daily basis? Why do we have so many ranges of sizes, holding onto the anticipation that we might get a deathly flu and actually suck ourselves into that dress one more time? Time for a wardrobe overhaul. Toss, donate, sell, or give clothes away to friends. Then replace them with clothes that fit you currently. And if by chance you do end up losing some inches later, do this again. But stop the madness of this mind game we play with ourselves every time we look in that closet and see those ultra skinny jeans looking back at us.

I owned a pair of size twenty-six Parasuco jeans once. They cost me $200 and were the bomb! I think I fit into them for one week of my life, when I was in a really unhealthy place with food, my body, and my exercise regimen. Every time I opened my closet, staring at me with their denim washes were the perfect jeans — haunting me and almost teasing me. They looked back at me like, "You are soooooo fat now, you will never be good enough to wear me," when in reality, I was a very healthy and very amazing size twenty-nine. So why did I keep telling myself that in order to be worthy and better, I would one day need to fit into those insanely skinny jeans again?

I gave them away. And replaced them with an equally amazing $200 pair of True Religion jeans in a size twenty-nine, which fit like a glove and really showed off how awesome my ass was. Letting go of the past and not letting those jeans define my self-worth anymore was the best thing I could have done. I finally embraced the body I had. This doesn't mean I still don't strive to one day be a size twenty-eight perhaps.

But when that day comes, I will head out on that shopping trip with my credit card in hand. In the meantime, I will wear clothes that fit and make me feel amazing. So fill your closet with kick-ass clothing that fits you now and shows off your amazing curves and edges!

**Focus on general health and on being free of disease or illness.** When we think about what our body actually does for us, instead of just seeing the shell of the exterior, we can see the bigger picture. I once had a breast cancer scare, and that was enough to shock me into being more careful about how I treat my body. I was more aware of the chemicals I was putting into and on my body. I had more gratitude for being able to move and breathe each day. Think about how you feel when you have a really bad flu. You just want to be healthy again. All you want is to get through day-to-day tasks again with ease instead of being bedridden. You just want to be able to eat a proper meal again without throwing it up. Then, when we get better, we forget that feeling of just wanting to be able to live, of caring less about how much fat we have to lose and more about just being able to live our lives with ease and enjoyment.

**Buy the best bras and undergarments.** This sounds crazy, but have you ever really, truly been properly fitted for a bra? It will change your life to actually wear the right size. I was walking around in a 34B for years. It pinched, made me uncomfortable, and could actually put me in a bad mood. Then I hit one of those higher end lingerie stores, where they do a proper fitting for you — they are skilled and trained in this. My consultant was a kind older woman who proceeded to tell me that I was in fact a 36C — far from what I had been sticking myself into for over a decade. Well, she then brought me the cutest, sexiest, most amazing 36C. I put it on, and I actually believed for a moment that I could either hit the Victoria's Secret runway or run the country. Or both! It changed the way I carried myself through my day, and it changed how I felt about my body. It fit properly, so I could then be comfortable in my own skin. It's amazing how good you can feel when you have something under your clothes that helps you embrace your body instead of making you want to rip if off the moment you get in the house at the end of the day.

**Get naked.** Now this doesn't necessarily mean hitting up the closest nude beach. But have you ever been naked in public and just stripped down? I was in Las Vegas at Caesars Palace a few years back, in their amazing spa. I went the first day and was super covered up.

I saw that clothing was optional — the space was all women, not co-ed. But I would still wrap my towel around myself everywhere I went, which meant I wasn't fully experiencing it all since I was so hung up on my body (which was at the time ultra lean and amazing). I went back on day two, and there was a large group of European ladies in their fifties. They saw me scurry from room to room with my tightly wrapped towel. We were all in the sauna together at one point, and one very nice woman watched as I carefully kept myself wrapped up. In her beautiful Italian accent, she said, "My darling, if I had a body like yours, I would be walking around the casino and Vegas strip with no clothes on." She was telling me to stop the madness! I actually let the towel go, and I swear it was a moment I felt I could take on the world. I remember sitting and chatting with all of these women about the female body and how, in Europe, it is viewed so much differently. Nudity is not as sexual; it's more just a way of life to embrace your body and your shape. I have tried to take this with me even years later. I will go topless at the hotel pool and not give a crap (if it is a topless pool, that is — let's look for signs). I will not worry so much about being naked during a massage. It's just a body, and no matter what the shape, size, flaws, or curves . . . it is amazing and should never been hidden or be a source of embarrassment.

**Embrace other women's bodies to see the good in your own.** I love seeing my friends, in all their shapes and sizes. I love seeing a woman with huge curves. I love seeing how different we all are, so I make it a point to not only see the amazing traits and differences in other women, but to compliment them and tell them as well. My daughter taught me this. From a young age, she would tell everyone she met about the good qualities that she saw in them. Maybe I taught her this indirectly, or maybe she just sees the pain in people's eyes and knows they need to hear something good for once (and coming from a child, it's from a genuine place). I now take this with me wherever I go. I was at the airport once and I saw a lady with the most amazing body shape. She wasn't tiny or lean by any means; it was more about how she just whisked herself through the airport with such confidence. I just had to hunt her down and say something to her. I saw her in line at Starbucks and went up to her and said, "I just wanted to say I love the aura you present, it's so stunning to see such a beautiful person — and I am straight and not hitting on you, FYI." Her eyes lit up, and she was so thankful. We actually sat next to each other while waiting for the plane. She mentioned that she was heading to California for a job interview and was not feeling super confident. My words really sat with her, and she was ready to kick some interview ass after my comments. It made me feel better about myself and my own appearance to comment and compliment someone else. When I notice how well others carry themselves, I, too, want to have that same aura and confidence in my own swagger.

**Learn to own your compliments.** For a whole month, I complimented as many women as possible. I wanted to see how they reacted. Many would downplay my compliments or not accept them. If I said, "Wow, you are really looking amazing in those jeans," they would assume it was thanks to the jeans, not their ass in it! I would comment on how beautiful their hair was, and they would respond by saying too bad they weren't ten pounds lighter. For every compliment, there was always some negative. Not one woman just said, "Thank you." We feel this need to come back with something terrible about ourselves, but who is that making feel better? We make the person delivering the kind words feel bad, and we make ourselves feel bad as well. Take the compliment, and don't overthink it or downplay it. Own your shit! It's not being cocky or arrogant to agree, "Yes, I kick ass!"

I want you to close your eyes. Just take a moment to imagine what it would be like if we truly saw ourselves for the amazing beings we are. Keep your eyes closed and as you breathe in deeply, I want you to feel the air filling up your amazing body. As you exhale, long and slow, I want you to let go of all the negativity you feel towards your body. Breathe in and think of some amazing things you are thankful for about your body. Things you love about your body. Exhale and let go of any flaws you dwell on, any feelings of insecurity. Now just sit with a natural breath and with your eyes still softly closed. I want you to imagine loving your body without judgements, without the inner critic. I want you to say to yourself softly, "I embrace every curve, edge, line, and asset on my body." "I embrace me." "I am empowered to love and rock the shit out of this body that I am lucky to have." "I am going to open my eyes and see the amazing being and the body that i am and have." Now open your eyes. And be so blessed to have such an amazing body to embrace! Find that feeling of full acceptance, embracing yourself to the moon and back, and you will find the body you have always wanted — because it's been right in front of you the whole time.

*When I was young I thought I should be built more like an athlete - long and lean - not with a womanly figure. But then people my age started coming up to me, saying "I love you because of the way you look." They could relate to me. That was really motivating. So I learned to be proud of my curves and to embrace my large boobs and my butt. I'm also about loving who you are and realizing you're beautiful.*

~ SERENA WILLIAMS

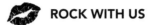
## 💋 ROCK WITH US

Snap a pic a pic of how you are embracing your body!! Maybe make it one of those funky boudoir shoots, G-rated please! It can also just be you rockin' your new jeans – anything! **INSPIRE** and hashtag us at **#kissmycurvyassets**

## NOTES

_____

_____

_____

_____

_____

_____

_____

_____

_____

_____

_____

_____

_____

_____

_____

_____

_____

_____

# CHAPTER 20

# GET INSPIRATION FROM CELEBRITIES WHO OWN THEIR SHAPE AND BODY IDEALS

*There are so many glamorous actresses, but in the real world, nobody looks like that. I want to inspire girls who don't think they're cool or pretty.*

~ REBEL WILSON

In a world filled with women conforming to the ideals and norms set out by society, it's both inspiring and empowering to see some celebrities who own their shit and not feel the pressure to fit in that cookie-cutter mold. I wanted to feature each and every one of these kick-ass, body-positive hotties because they truly embrace what makes them different or unique. Thanks to their power and voice, we can stand even stronger in this movement to change the way we as women see ourselves and our bodies.

I was able to fit in five great stories of celebs who lift me up with their attitudes and mindset. When I compiled my list of inspirational women that are celebrities, I realized I clearly had over fifty amazing ladies, but the book could only be so long. I have to give honorable mentions to those who didn't make my top five picks, but I just couldn't leave out them of this chapter.

**Rebel Wilson** has made her mark in Hollywood, and this stunning actress has revealed that paving her own way in the industry and sticking to her own beauty standards have actually helped her further her career. She told *Cosmopolitan*, "I feel really lucky to be the body type I am."[36] Go, Rebel!

**Mindy Kaling** admits to struggling with being a body-positive celebrity and to having a "complicated relationship" with her body, but she also doesn't see the point in depriving herself to lose weight. That is why she makes my list — you go girl!

**Melissa McCarthy** has to make the list of honorable mentions. She told *Redbook*, "Give me your best punch in the face, and I'll take that punch, rather than have my kid feel bad about herself." She also said, "There's an epidemic in our country of girls and women feeling bad about themselves based on what 0.5% of the human race looks like. My message is that as long as everybody's healthy, enjoy and embrace whatever body type you have."[37] Melissa is paving the way for future generations with her body-positive attitude! Love it!

**Tina Fey** makes us laugh with everything she does, and she was quoted as saying, "If you retain nothing else, always remember the most important rule of beauty, which is: Who cares?"[38] Love this attitude, Tina! Let go of caring; the rat-race is tiring!

**Christina Aguilera** has taken so much heat for the fuller curves she sports these days. But the former *The Voice judge* once said, "You can never be too much of anything. You can never be too perfect, too thin, too curvy, too voluptuous, this, that [every] female in this business at one time or another has had criticism." This pop icon has perfected the art of ignoring the body-shamers, adding, "As long as I'm happy in my own skin, that's all I need, that's all the confirmation I need. I'm happy where I am."[39] Go, Christina!

**Selena Gomez** has dealt with tons of body-shamers recently, and she posted on her Instagram, "The beauty myth- an obsession with physical perfection that traps modern woman in an endless cycle of hopelessness, self-consciousness, and self-hatred as she tries to fulfill society's impossible definition of flawless beauty." She also emphasized, "I chose to take care of myself because I want to, not to prove anything to anyone." Wind in her sails. Boom!

I seriously need to be best friends with **Adele**, as her outlook on her body and body ideals motivates me and inspires me. She once said in an article for the *Huffington Post,* "I've seen people where it rules their lives, who want to be thinner or have bigger boobs, and how it wears them down . . . And I don't want that in my life. I have insecurities, of course, but I don't hang out with anyone who points them out to me."[40] This woman ROCKS!

**Kate Winslet** admits to struggling with body image, and also aims to ensure that her daughter doesn't. On *People.com*, she described an exercise she does with her young daughter. "I stand in front of the mirror and say to Mia, 'We are so lucky we have a shape. We're so lucky we're curvy. We're so lucky that we've got good bums.' And she'll say, 'Mummy, I know, thank God.'" [41] Go, Mama Kate!

Who doesn't love sweetheart **Drew Barrymore**? And she had to make my list of honorable body-positive mentions after she commented to *InStyle Magazine*, "I am who I am and I just don't have a bikini body . . . I don't even have a one-piece body anymore! But I am loving the long rash guard, board-shorts look." [42] Drew, you are amazing! You kick ass!

**Jennifer Aniston** also had to make the list thanks to her long experience with societal and social media madness. She said in a *Vogue* interview, "I don't think it's getting much better. I think the problem is the tabloids and the gossip columns taking the human body and putting it in a category." She explained, "They're either fat-shaming, or body-shaming, or childless-shaming. It's a weird obsession that people have, and I don't understand exactly why they need to take people who are out there to entertain you, and rip them apart and bully them? Why are we teaching young women this? It's incredibly damaging." [43] Amen to that, Jen!

**Kelly Clarkson** wins my "screw-you society" award. The *American Idol* winner discussed one of the darkest periods in her career during an interview with *Attitude magazine*. "When I was really skinny, I wanted to kill myself," she said. "I was miserable, like, inside and out, for four years of my life. But, no one cared, because aesthetically, you make sense." [44] Kelly no longer conforms to societal ideals, and she also ensures her daughters can do the same. "Even from a young age, I think you should instill that people, your children, should always stand up for themselves or speak out when something is wrong . . . I think if we start it at that young age, and you start molding people and growing to (sic) these very elevated individuals that help elevate society." [45] Kelly is paving the way for our future girls to define their body ideals on their own terms.

**Katy Perry**, you had me at *I Kissed A Girl*. And your body image tops my list of game changers in the body ideals world. Katy told *People. com*, "My body's changing and I'm like, 'It's winter, and I'm like hibernating. I'm storing the foods, I'm thick, I'm happy about it . . . There are things that I wear that sometimes I [don't] feel like I look great in them, but you don't have to be skin and bones."[46] Katy not only promotes being yourself (since you are an original and the world would be very boring if we were all the same), she also loves being weird, standing out, and not being the cookie-cutter traditional rock-star. Just be you. We love you, Katy!

**Demi Lovato** has openly struggled with bipolar disorder, drug and alcohol addictions, and an eating disorder. "Sometimes when I'm having bad body image issue days, I remind myself that I'd rather live in freedom from my eating disorder than worry about what people think about my body," she wrote for *People.com*. "I am more than a number and a jean size," Lovato continued.[47] In 2018, she posted a pic of herself in a bathing suit on Instagram with the following comment, "So, I'm insecure about my legs in this picture but I'm posting it because I look so happy and this year, I've decided I'm letting go of my perfectionism and embracing freedom from self-criticism." She continued, "Learning to love my body the way it is is challenging but life changing. Today I'm feeling strong. You all can do it too. It IS possible. Thank you God for this new chapter in my life. #EDrecovery #happyAF." And I am happy AF she is embracing her body and sharing this with us women!

**Serena Williams** gets my "best badass body-acceptance athlete" award. In an ESPN interview with her friend Common, Serena stated, "There was a time when I didn't feel incredibly comfortable about my body because I felt like I was too strong . . . I had to take a second and think, 'Who says I'm too strong? This body has enabled me to be the greatest player that I can be. And now my body is in style, so I'm feeling good about it. Like, I'm finally in style! It took a while to get there."

She continued, "I'm just really thankful for the way I was brought up by my mum and my dad to give me that confidence. I could have been discouraged, and I wouldn't be as great as I was because I would have done different exercises or I would have done different things. I totally embrace who I am and what I am."[48] Strong, athletic, and a world-class athlete and woman! Thank you, Serena!

This list could go on and on, but I'd like to finally salute the Goddess, the queen . . . **Miss Oprah Winfrey**! I may cry thinking about all this woman has endured in terms of body-shaming, body image issues, and just learning to love the awesome being she is. On her website *Oprah.com*, she said, "After spending the past ten weeks in class with Eckhart Tolle, studying his book *A New Earth*, I know for sure that I am not my body. I feel more connected to consciousness, or soul, or inner spirit — whatever you choose to name the formless being that is the essence of who we are. I think of all the years I've wasted hating my-self fat, wanting myself thin. Feeling guilty about every croissant, then giving up carbs, then fasting, then dieting, then worrying when I wasn't dieting, then eating everything I wanted until the next diet. Wasted time, abhorring the thought of trying on clothes, wondering what was going to fit, what number the scale would say. All that energy I could have spent loving what is."[49] Drop the mic — we love you just the way you are, too! You get self-esteem, and you get self-esteem, and you get self-esteem!

Like I said, I wanted to spend so much more time featuring all of these women, but I stripped my final list down to just five women whom I use for inspiration. These women are paving the way for body acceptance and rocking what they have.

**Amy Schumer.** I could have written a whole book dedicated to just this woman and her insane amounts of self-love, body acceptance, and change of industry standards. Where do I even start with Amy? In a write-up in *People* magazine, the comedian joked, "I'm what Holly-wood calls 'very fat.'"[50] In *Trainwreck*, she was tricked into losing a few pounds to fit societal ideals. She commented, "I look very stupid skinny. My dumb head stays the same, but then my body, like, shrivels and [I] just look like . . . a Thanksgiving Day parade [balloon] of Tonya Harding . . . Nobody likes it. It's not cute on me."[51] Amy rocks being in her own skin, once saying in her Netflix special, "I feel very good in my own skin. I feel strong. I feel healthy. I do. I feel sexy." Let's talk about *I Feel Pretty*, the movie released in 2018, which is all about the body-positive movement and finally seeing the beauty in yourself, regardless of size, shape, make, or model. In the *LA Times* online, Amy was quoted saying, "I don't know that the country really has an appetite to hear the story of a white, blonde woman with a belly."[52] She also admitted, "I get it." She also wants women to feel "empowered to live up to their full potential" — to not be held back by the fear of being perceived as fat or ugly. In her Netflix special *The Leather Special*, she talks about the media. "They photographed me once, and this was the headline: 'Schumer buys pastry so she can work out.' Kind of mean, right? No, they hit the nail right on the [expletive] head. That's what I do to work out. Before I work out, I go buy a scone, and then I slowly walk around a reservoir, and I eat it. My workouts are like a woman in hospice. Just, like, nibbling on a baked good, looking at the trees and the birds." At one point, Schumer admits she felt so bad about her appearance that she even attempted to get an eating disorder — a journey she said lasted all of two hours, when she realized she couldn't stand being hungry. "It's not worth it to me to live this life where I have to be really hungry."[51] Speaking of the trolls and body shamers, Schumer said, "I've been told I'm fat. I'm ugly. I've seen memes of me being the grossest woman in the world — me as Jabba the Hut. The fear is gone." "I just decided to believe my own hype," she explained. "If you think of the things you would say to your friends when they're having a bad day — why don't you let yourself take care of yourself like that? I understand that that's really scary and makes you feel really vulnerable." Schumer has talked about *I Feel Pretty* and how she really wanted to be sure she showed her body on-screen the way it truly is. There's one scene in which her character — post head-bump — decides to compete in a bikini contest alongside a half dozen statuesque women who are stick thin. "In post, they asked me if I wanted to retouch anything, and I was like, 'What? No,'" she said. "I love it. I think I look sexy and strong."[51] Body acceptance and Amy go hand-in-hand, and I will close this blurb talking about the pic from the 2016 *Pirelli* calendar shoot in which she posed almost nude and in her full raw body. "That photo got so much positive feedback. Somebody photoshopped it right next to a picture of Aphrodite in the same position and our bodies were pretty similar," she notes. "So it was kind of cool to be like, 'this is what (beauty) used to be before it was the image of a starving actress model who doesn't eat as regularly as they would like'." She smiles. "I'm proud of it."[52] Amy, keep being you — you are fuckin' fabulous!

**Ashley Graham**. Another pioneer in the body-positive world, someone who embodies the "fitness comes in all shapes and sizes movement," is Miss Ashley Graham . . . DROOL! "When I was seventeen or eighteen-years-old," says model Ashley Graham, "I was doing a group shot for this really big campaign, and one girl, who was probably a size two or four, said to me, 'Did you actually get paid for this job?' I remember thinking, 'She's asking me that because I'm fat.'" Graham, now twenty-nine-years-old, still runs into that model (whom, taking the high road, she refuses to name). "She's always friendly and nice," says Graham. "I think she forgot she said it. But it's one of those things I'll never forget."[53] A decade later, Graham has proven not only that she can and should get paid, but also that she can — and will — change the whole damn world. She was the first size-sixteen model ever to be featured on the cover of the *Sports Illustrated's* swimsuit issue. Graham didn't always feel so confident; in fact, she nearly gave up modelling out of the fear of being rejected. Her mom told her, "You're there for a reason. Your body is there to change the lives of people."[54] Thanks,

Mama Graham! Ashley transformed how she viewed herself and began posting selfies to her now almost seven million followers on social media. Ashley did an amazing *Ted Talk* speech in which she talked about the power of self-acceptance and her problem with being labeled a plus-sized model. This is how her talk started: "Back fat, I see you popping over my bra today. But that's alright — I'm going to choose to love you. Thick thighs, you're just so sexy, you can't stop rubbing each other. That's alright, I'm going to keep you. And cellulite, I have not forgotten about you — I'm going to choose to love you, even though you want to take over my whole bottom half."[55] BOW DOWN, Miss Graham! I just love this! She went on to say that being labelled a "plus-sized model" made her feel like she was an outsider in the fashion world. She is like my movement — she is pioneering the way to break free of the molds. In her Ted Talk she also said, "I felt free once I realized I was never going to fit in the mold that society wanted me to fit in. I'm never going to be perfect enough for an industry that defines perfection from the outside in... rolls, curves, cellulite — all of it. I love every part of me."[56] Women everywhere, say thank you to Ashley — preach on my curvy sister. Perfect is overrated and you are a goddess!

**Jennifer Lawrence.** Want a positive body image? This gal rocks it! She has been defined as the "normal" body, but she said, "I would like us to make a new normal body type." Jennifer says that she works out more than most normal people, but that society has gotten us "so used to underweight that when you are normal weight it's like, 'OMG she's so curvy!'" J-law doesn't diet; in fact, her comments on embracing a diet-free life were, "You have to look past it — you look how you look, and be comfortable. What are you going to do? Be hungry every single day to make other people happy? That's just dumb." Jennifer speaks openly about hoping we can stop these judgements of others, emphasizing it's not funny to point out if we think people are ugly or fat. It's so inspiring that she knows younger girls look up to her and she needs to be a healthy body image role model, if not for herself, then for the younger generation. She believes that strong is the new skinny. "I'm a woman that's living in this world of everybody telling everyone how they should look and what they should be eating and how people can lose this much weight this fast, and it just kind of overwhelms our senses. If I could just make the tiniest bit of difference in getting rid of that because it is so annoying, I would love that."[57] She has also worked hard to help eliminate the word "fat", saying it should be "illegal" to call someone fat on TV. Keep kicking ass, Jennifer!

**Lady Gaga.** The world can be such a mean and nasty place. A while back, Gaga posted pictures of herself — in the raw, no makeup, and in her underwear. The media had been criticizing her for gaining twenty-five pounds. Her gesture was surprisingly simple and subtle — she posted the photos under the caption, "Bulimia and Anorexia since I was fifteen."[58] Wow! This woman was admitting to struggling with such a tough disease for decades, and the media should be ashamed for contributing to it! Then she invited her enormous fan base to join her in a "Body Revolution" and to show the world what their bodies really look like. She invited women everywhere to speak out about their eating disorders, body-shaming, and body-hatred. I get tears thinking about the impact she has made by being so raw and real, inviting others to do the same. It's insane to see the media post before-and-after weight gain pictures of a star and then comment on whether it was acceptable or not, like it's their place to even have an opinion. Gaga actually justified her weight gain at first, blaming frequent Italian restaurant meals. "I love eating pizza and pasta, I'm a New York Italian girl," she explained to interviewers. She then stopped justifying and told her followers, "Seeing you post photos of things on your bodies and in your minds that you feel society tells you you should be ashamed of. You are showing them you have no shame. You are brave, strong, and accepting not only of yourself, but of others through your experiences. You are proud to be born this way, and brave in your vulnerability with this community. My weight / loss / gain since I was child has tormented me.

No amount of help has ever healed my pain about it. But YOU have. Love, Gaga"[59] Then, in the *Super Bowl* halftime show, Gaga showed insane talent, with high-flying acrobatics, a parade of hits, and her commanding stage presence. Sadly, this was all tragically overlooked because many just focused on her body. Gaga is insanely fit, but of course the body-shamers criticized her for not having their definition of a "perfect" figure. One hater wrote, "Her stomach is literally hanging over her shorts and looks horrible." Another picked apart her stomach, saying it was "flabby" and "protruding slightly." If you saw the pictures, you would cringe at that comment — her stomach was amazing! In an honest and powerful Instagram post, Gaga told fans (and haters) she is proud of her body and encourages everyone else to embrace themselves, despite all the noise (I would have told them to bite me, but you go, Gaga!). "I heard my body is a topic of conversation, so I wanted to say, I'm proud of my body and you should be proud of yours too. I could give you a million reasons why you don't need to cater to anyone or anything to succeed. Be you, and be relentlessly you. That's the stuff of champions."[60] (Bow down!) She has brought attention to the negativity surrounding the body-shamers, but has also reminded us to "just be real, be us" . . . and for that, she is a body-positive and self-acceptance icon! I freakin' love this woman!

**Tyra Banks.** Last on the list, but first in my heart for this whole body-positive movement, is Miss Tyra. A-MAZING can't even sum up how I define this woman. Ms. Banks has spoken about her battles with weight, body image, and self-esteem for decades. She helps support teens struggling with their weight and is so inspiring with her body acceptance. "I've had some of my girls talk about their weight, and I actually talk to them honestly about it," says Banks, who mentors teens through her foundation. "There's one thing you can do, which is say, 'You're great, you're great, you're great,' which makes them feel good in that moment when you're talking to them," Tyra explains. "So what I tell my girls is, health is important, and we need to get our shapes in shape

— not looking like somebody else."[61] Over a decade ago, she went on television and told her haters to "kiss my ass" when talking about some photos that had surfaced of her on the beach. In the paparazzi shots, the star was standing on the shore in a one-piece suit showing off her amazing and curvy hourglass figure. The tabloids were filled with insanity and mean people who captioned the pics "Thigh-ra Banks," "America's Next Top Waddle", and "Tyra Porkchops." Even with this brutal scrutiny, Tyra fired back at her haters and shamers in a teary-eyed speech: "I love my mama. She has helped me to be a strong woman so I can overcome these kind of attacks, but if I had lower self-esteem, I would probably be starving myself right now. But that's exactly what is happening to other women all over this country. So I have something to say to all of you that have something nasty to say about me or other women who are built like me… women whose names you know, women whose names you don't, women who've been picked on, women whose husbands put them down, women at work or girls in school — I have one thing to say to you: Kiss my fat ass."[62] I can remember cheering along from my sofa at home along as the audience cheered. I can remember being teary-eyed myself, but so proud of her message. Tyra told People, "I've made millions of dollars with the body I have, so where's the pain in that? If I was in pain, I would have dieted."[63] She is a mentor to other models, and also to regular women everywhere! We love your assets, Miss Tyra! You go, girl!

When I first wrote the rough draft for this chapter, it was over 25,000 words. I could have included so many amazing body-positive and uplifting celebs — perhaps it will be my next book! I was able to narrow it down and touch on some of the great ones, but had to cut out so many inspiring stories. Let's take a page from these celebrities, who are in the battlefield and on the front lines of body-shaming and have society ideals being forced down their throats. They are choosing to fight back, stand up, take back control of their ideals, and rock the shit out of their bodies!

*Don't waste so much time thinking about how much you weigh. There is no more mind-numbing, boring, idiotic, self-destructive diversion from the fun of living.*

~ MERYL STREEP

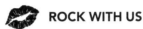 **ROCK WITH US**

Share a link or a screengrab of an influencer or celeb that amazes you! Help us all find new and inspiring women who show **#kissmycurvyassets** how to **ROCK OUR ASSETS**! Be sure to tag the celeb too, so they know they are helping other women kick-ass in the body-loving department.

## NOTES

_____

_____

_____

_____

_____

_____

_____

_____

_____

_____

_____

_____

## NOTES

_____

_____

_____

_____

_____

_____

_____

_____

_____

_____

_____

_____

_____

_____

_____

_____

_____

_____

_____

_____

_____

_____

_____

_____

_____

# READY TO ROCK

*I love to see a young girl go out and grab the world by the lapels. Life's a bitch. You've got to go out and kick ass.*

~ MAYA ANGELOU

Lies! We have been made to believe outright lies for years and even decades. As children, we are shown images of the female body that are out of reach or even imaginary. As young teens, we are bombarded with this idea that our bodies equal our self-worth. As young women, we buy into this concept that less food and more exercise will give us the dream body that media keeps pushing on us. As women, we put such high attachment and value to the number on the scale or the size of our jeans. All of this leads to comparison, judgement, self-hate, obsession, and a downward spiral that results in mass destruction of female egos everywhere.

But wait! What if we took back this control? What if we took the tools in this book, even just from one or two chapters, and started to shift our way of thinking? What if we started to change the outlook we have about our bodies? How would it feel if we embraced, accepted, highlighted, and rocked the shit out of the bodies we have, and in turn finally achieved those long-term fitness and wellness goals? Who is ready to join this movement of women all over the world owning the bodies they have and kicking ass in this world, regardless of the norms or ideals? Creating our own ideals, molding our bodies to be what we want them to be. Letting go of the self-bullying or abuse. Freeing ourselves from the insanity and madness.

Thirty-three billion dollars. This is the amount of money sunk into an industry that wants us to keep hating our bodies. This industry wants us to continue the rat race of never finding self-acceptance. It feeds off of our insecurities and desperation. If we own our shit, they lose and we win! We will no longer listen to their lies and nonsense.

The female body has surely evolved through the years, and social norms have also changed accordingly and will continue to do so. Despite everything, one thing is for sure — we women are powerful, amazing beings. We get to control how we feel and how we look. We have always had this control and power; we have just been giving it away. The time has now come to own it and reclaim our power.

In this book, we covered strategies to help us embrace, highlight, and rock the shit out of our bodies. It comes down to something so simple: change our mindset and lifestyle:

| CURRENT MINDSET & LIFESTYLE | REFRAMED MINDSET & LIFESTYLE |
|---|---|
| • Self body-shaming | • Finding body positivity |
| • Negative self-talk | • Empowering self-talk |
| • Crash/fad/or extreme diets with harsh rebounds | • Sustainable, nourishing nutrition plan for life |
| • Impossible workout regimens causing overtraining | • Exercise as a form of fun — not punishment |
| • Being a slave to the scale and numbers | • Freedom from the numbers game |
| • Body hate and loathing | • Self-acceptance and self-love |
| • Fighting our natural body shape | • Embracing all of our curves and as-sets |
| • Worrying what others think of us | • Being free to own our shit and release the hold of others' opinions |
| • A cluttered negative mind | • Positive thinking and fresh mindset |
| • Our negative self-esteem affecting quality of life, career, and relationships | • Happy body = finding happiness with all aspects of life, career, relationships. You can't find success until you are happy from within. |

Dizzy from everything we covered, unsure of what to do or where to start? Let's recap this book and all of the principles to help you rock the shit out of your body with ease:

## LORI'S K.I.S.S (KEEP IT SIMPLE SEXY) PRINCIPLES

**1. Create your own damn body ideals** and screw what society says or shows you!

**2. Don't go it alone** — search for some other badass babes to join your girl-squad and all of you can rock your bodies together!

**3. Own the shit out of your social media accounts**, and never let what someone else posts affect your own body image.

**4. Train your mindset above anything else, and the exterior results just freakin' happen!** Think you are hot AF, and you better believe you will be hot AF!.

**5. Tell the scale to *fuck off*!** It has no power over your self-worth, so time to say BUH-BYE!

**6. Fad diets, extremes, and fitness programming insanity — you are dead to me!** Time to BREAK IT OFF!

**7. Give fewer shits about what others think of you.** You do you, Boo!

**8. Remember your 4 S's** - Self (Love, Acceptance, Esteem, and Care).

**9. Don't forget to use the 3 M's** (Meditation, Mantras, and Motivation).

**10. Have a lot of sex, and ensure that you ORGASM A SHIT TON!** I repeat — CUM OFTEN!

**11. Stop holding on to past beliefs or fuck-ups.** LET THAT SHIT GO!

**12. The monster of jealousy or comparison will kill ya**, so stop that comparison game and focus on watering your own green grass!

13. **Try your best to fuel yourself with the best nutrition (most of the time)**, eat foods you enjoy, and make a plan that works for your real life. If all else fails, listen to your body and give it what it tells you it needs.

14. **Exercise doesn't have to be beast-mode.** Do things you enjoy and that you WANT TO DO! Move those assets how you want to!

15. **Stop setting impossible goals, stop focusing only on numbers (like your weight)**, and start small to find baby steps that are sustainable in the long-term.

16. **Remember your H.A.T - Hormones, Adrenals, and Thyroid, oh my!** Those internal systems are the control centre for what is going to happen externally.

17. **Hey potty mouth, lose those swear words: failure, starvation, perfection, deprivation, transformation, and even the word diet.** They aren't serving you!

18. **Be the wiser older woman and show younger ladies the way to owning what they got!** You are a mentor, so if you own it, they will follow suit!

19. **Embrace what God gave ya** — own every inch of those curves and assets!

20. **Join the celebrity movement to break free of those society ideals and norms** and rock the shit we all got!

Print that list off — study it, use it, own it, and I promise you . . . in the end, it will have you ROCKIN' THE SHIT OUT OF YOUR BODY!

Thank you for reading this book. Thank you for taking the time to look for other ways to find that body acceptance and long-term body love. Thank you for knowing it was time for a change, time for a movement in which we, as women, can come together and finally give up this charade of trying to fit into a mold we were never meant to fit into in the first place.

If you could take just one thing away from this book, I would love for it to be this: You deserve to love your body. You deserve to look at all of the edges, inches, pounds, curves, and lines of your body and FREAKING ROCK IT! You deserve to release these handcuffs we have all been in for so long, this prison that says our body has anything to do with our worth. Fitness and women's bodies come in such an amazing variety of shapes and sizes. You are allowed to own what you have, rock what you want, and kick ass being the amazing woman that you are.

I get it, you want to have a hot body. But if you stood back and truly looked at yourself inside and out, embraced all that you have, you would see that staring back at you is already the canvas of a beautiful work of art. Being hot AF means owning your power, owning your body — scars, cellulite, freckles, muscle tone, everything! Please don't change — don't transform . . . be you! Be real and keep doing you! You freakin' rock!

I don't want this book to end. You see, this book took me twenty-seven years to bring to light. This book is an explosion of emotions stemming from the sadness and the madness I have seen in the eyes of so many broken women, myself included. But this book is here, this movement has begun to rise, and although this is the last chapter, this is not the end. This is your time to write your new chapter. Take your body, every inch of it, and create what you want to create. Be who you want to be. Share this experience and story with other women everywhere — younger generations, friends, coworkers, any woman who may also need someone to reach out to them and reassure them that it is safe, more than okay, and absolutely amazing to be themselves, own their body, and rock the God-given assets they've been blessed with!

*There is more to life than the calories I consume and the sessions I spend sweating at the gym. I define my own body ideals. I choose the way I want to look and feel. My curves and edges are amazing just as they are, so I will highlight and embrace them, and anyone who has a problem with it can . . . KISS MY CURVY ASSETS!*

~ LORI MORK

## ACKNOWLEDGMENT

Where do I even begin . . .

Thank you to women everywhere. Thank you for those who helped strengthen me with inspiring stories of breakdowns and break-throughs. Thank for you sharing your struggles and helping me to see that with all sadness and loss, we can find happiness and gains.

I am beyond lucky to have the most amazing best friend in the world, Patti Lewis. You are the most inspiring woman I know. Your friendship is something I am beyond blessed to have, and even through the distance and miles, I feel your strength, inspiration, and power with me daily. Patti, you are the Thelma to my Louise!

I also have the most kick ass group of a girl squad a gal could ask for. They make me laugh my ass off and show me that wine and insane girls' nights trump a tight ass any day! Kristin, Kaley, Brigette, Patty, Christina, Sheri, Tera, Sarah, Jericho, Kindra, Andrea, Ruth, Kim. And the list goes on and on - you are my rock, and possibly the people who will be responsible for sending me to rehab for my wine consumption — but with good intentions! Lol!

Sixteen years ago, I got the best gift anyone could ask for, a baby girl: Brooklyn. A girl who has blossomed into the most beautiful teenager. Thank you for showing me that I too am worthy of receiving and partaking in the proper self-love I deserve. For bringing to awareness the mind-boggling and skewed perceptions of the media. For giving me the courage and determination I needed to fight for this change in order to pave the way for you, and younger women everywhere. In life, the most important thing I want for you, my dear Brooklyn, is to see your inner beauty and celebrate it, while, and allow it to not be connected to the external body focus that society pushes on us.

# ACKNOWLEDGMENT

Twelve years ago, I got another best gift anyone could ask for, a baby boy, Beckham. A boy who shows me that stereotypes do not define us. When you are a boy, your favorite color can be pink, and your favorite sport can be ballet. Beckham, having you as my son was just what I needed to show what it looks and feels like to be someone who accepts everyone, someone who sees everyone for their true authentic selves, and just has fun being his best self. What a lucky mom I am!

I have been in this crazy fitness industry as a trainer and coach for twenty-seven years, and without this experience, I could not have had the knowledge, experience, stories, and scars from seeing so many of my clients' struggles and triumphs. My clients are my inspiration, they are my guinea pigs on this journey to find the answer to the question I have always had: How can I own what I want in terms of body ideals, and rock the shit out of them? Each of you being broken down has enabled me to find ways to help you repair, reprogram, and retake control of female well-being worldwide.

When searching for a publisher, it was fate, I believe, that brought me to GBR Publishing. Ky-Lee, soul sister, guide, juggler of so much - you are superwoman and this is just the beginning of our collaborations. Thank you to Anya-Milana, Tania, and Sara, my editors, who had the toughest job in the world dissecting my mumbo-jumbo of words bringing them together as this book. To be the editing police when I went overboard with !!!!!!! or BOLD COMMENTS. To reel me in just enough, but allow me my voice, my sassiness, swear words, and my raw, real honesty of words. To Sar, thanks for designing a bad-ass cover!

This book was something I dreamed of as a child. I thought it would take flight as something fitness related, but I had no idea the need for it. The want for it. The cry for help for it. It was time to deliver something that could finally help us all embrace, highlight, and rock the shit out of our curves and assets.

Last but not least, my body. Yes, I am thanking my thunder thighs, I am thanking that big chunky-bum of mine. Thank you body, for all of the ups and downs you have taken me through over the decades. I have not been all that nice to you, but that has, and is, changing. Thank you body - for putting up with my shit and sticking around, with the bumps, bruises, and scars to prove it. But in the end you are my body, and I am gonna ROCK THE SHIT OUT OF YOU! Blessed to have you body!!!!!! Thanks for helping me write this book!

xoxo,

Lori

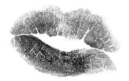

## ENDNOTES

1. Howard, J., & Ginsburg, A. (Writer and Videographer). "The history of the 'ideal' woman and where that has left us." *CNN*, March 9, 2018. https://www.cnn.com/2018/03/07/health/body-image-history-of-beauty-explainer-intl/index.html

2. Women's Body Image and BMI: 100 Years in the US. (n.d.). Retrieved from https://www.rehabs.com/explore/womens-body-image-and-bmi

3. Howard, J., & Ginsburg, A. (Writer and Videographer). "The history of the 'ideal' woman and where that has left us." *CNN*, March 9, 2018. https://www.cnn.com/2018/03/07/health/body-image-history-of-beauty-explainer-intl/index.html

4. Dreisbach, S. "Shocking Body-Image News: 97% of Women Will Be Cruel to Their Bodies Today." *Glamour*, February 11, 2011. https://www.glamour.com/story/shocking-body-image-news-97-percent-of-women-will-be-cruel-to-their-bodies-today

5. Allen, M. "This Dove Report Reveals Shocking Results About Women's Body Confidence." *Cosmopolitan*, March 16, 2018. https://www.cosmopolitan.com/style-beauty/beauty/news/a60373/womens-body-confidence-declining/

6. Howard, J., & Ginsburg, A. (Writer and Videographer). "The history of the 'ideal' woman and where that has left us." *CNN*, March 9, 2018. https://www.cnn.com/2018/03/07/health/body-image-history-of-beauty-explainer-intl/index.html

7. "Children, Teens, Media, and Body Image." *Common Sense Media*, January 21, 2015. https://www.commonsensemedia.org/research/children-teens-media-and-body-image

8. Foster, C. "An Open Letter to the Media about "Ideal" Body Image." *Health Fitness Revolution*, August 2, 2016. http://www.healthfitnessrevolution.com/open-letter-media-ideal-body-image/

9. Nugent, P., M.S. "BODY-IMAGE IDEALS?" *PsychologyDictionary.com*, April 7, 2013. https://psychologydictionary.org/body-image-ideals/

10. Simmons, R. "How Social Media Is a Toxic Mirror." *Time*, August 19, 2016. http://time.com/4459153/social-media-body-image/

11. *Dictionary.com*. "Mindset." https://www.dictionary.com/browse/mindset

12. "A Short History of the Weighing Scale." *Withings*, September 30, 2011. https://blog.withings.com/2011/09/30/a-short-history-of-the-weighing-scale-2/

13. Freedman, M. "Fad Diets." *Encyclopedia.com*, 2004. https://www.encyclopedia.com/food/news-wires-white-papers-and-books/fad-diets

14. "Overview of Nutrition." *HealthCommunities.com*, (n.d.). http://www.healthcommunities.com/nutrition-basics/overview-of-nutrition

15. Rotchford, L. "Diets Through History: The Good, Bad, and Scary." *Health*, January 24, 2018. https://www.health.com/health/gallery/0,,20653382,00.html

16. "23 Exceptional Fad Diet Statistics." *HealthResearchFunding.org*, October 9, 2014. https://healthresearchfunding.org/23-exceptional-fad-diet-statistics/

17. *Merriam-Webster Dictionary*, s.v. "Self-acceptance." https://www.merriam-webster.com/dictionary/self-acceptance

18. "A Man Named Bad (Self Acceptance)." (n.d.). http://www.buddhanet.net/bt_50.htm

19. *Merriam-Webster Dictionary*, s.v. "Self-Love." https://www.merriam-webster.com/dictionary/self-love

20. *Merriam-Webster Dictionary*, s.v. "Self-Esteem." https://www.merriam-webster.com/dictionary/self-esteem

21. "What Self-Care Is - and What It Isn't." *PsychCentral.com*, August 14, 2016. https://psychcentral.com/blog/what-self-care-is-and-what-it-isnt-2/

22. Ulrich-Lai, Y.M., Christiansen, et al. Pleasurable behaviors reduce stress via brain reward pathways. *Proceedings of the National Academy of Sciences* 107, no. 47 (2010): 20529-24.

23. Ulrich-Lai, Y.M., Christiansen, A.M., Ostrander, M.M., Jones, A. A., Jones, K. R., Choi, D. C., Krause, E. G., Evanson, N. K., Furay, A. R., Davis, J. F., Solomon, M. B., de Kloet, A. D., Tamashiro, K. L., Sakai, R. R., Seeley, R. J., Woods, S. C., and Hermana, J. P. Pleasurable behaviors reduce stress via brain reward pathways. *Proceedings of the National Academy of Sciences* 107, no. 47 (2010): 20529-24.

24. Castleman, M. "Want to Prevent Colds? Have Sex Weekly." *Psychology Today online*, June 1, 2009. https://www.psychologytoday.com/ca/blog/all-about-sex/200906/want-prevent-colds-have-sex-weekly

25. Joi, Sarah. "8 Sexy Ways to Burn Calories." *Woman's Day online*, 2016. https://www.womansday.com/relationships/sex-tips/advice/a1922/8-sexy-ways-to-burn-calories-110923/

26. *Dictionary.com.* "Jealous." https://www.dictionary.com/browse/jealous

27. *Dictionary.com.* "Comparison." https://www.dictionary.com/browse/comparison

28. *Dictionary.com* "Insecurity." https://www.dictionary.com/browse/insecurity?s=t

29. Doran, G et al. (1981, November). There's a S.M.A.R.T. Way to Write Management's Goals and Objectives. Management Review. 35-36.

30. *Dictionary.com.* "Failure." https://www.dictionary.com/browse/failure?s=t

31. *Dictionary.com.* "Starvation." https://www.dictionary.com/browse/starvation?s=t

32. *Dictionary.com.* "Perfection." https://www.dictionary.com/browse/perfection?s=t

33. *Dictionary.com.* "Deprivation." https://www.dictionary.com/browse/deprivation?s=t

34. *Dictionary.com.* "Transformation." https://www.dictionary.com/browse/transformation?s=t

35. Legend, J. *All of Me.* New York: GOOD Music, 2013.

# ENDNOTES

36. Delbyck, C. "Rebel Wilson Feels 'Really Lucky' to Have Her Body Type." *Huffpost online*, November 30, 2015. https://www.huffingtonpost.ca/entry/rebel-wilson-body-type-cosmopolitan_us_565cc7a8e4b072e9d1c2fafd

37. Newman, J. "Melissa McCarthy Shares Her Ultimate Secret to Happiness in Redbook's April Issue." *Redbook online*, March 8, 2016. https://www.redbookmag.com/life/interviews/a42962/melissa-mccarthy-redbook-april-2016-cover-star/

38. Fey, T. *Bossypants*. Boston, MA: Little, Brown and Company, 2011. Retrieved from https://www.goodreads.com/quotes/1268998-12-the-most-important-rule-of-beauty-if-you-retain

39. Price, Lydia. "Christina Aguilera: 5 Times She was a Body Image Winner." *People.com*, August 14, 2015. https://people.com/celebrity/christina-aguileras-body-image-wins/

40. Markovinovic, M. "Adele Opens Up About Body Image and Why She Doesn't Let It Affect Her." *Huffpost online*, November 19, 2015. https://www.huffingtonpost.ca/2015/11/19/adele-body-image_n_8602262.html

41. Yagoda, M. "Kate Winslet Preaches Body Positivity to Daughter Mia: 'We Are So Lucky We Have a Shape.'" *People.com*, July 28, 2015. https://people.com/bodies/kate-winslet-body-image-issues-on-running-wild/

42. Apatoff, A. "Drew Barrymore: 'I Am Who I Am and I Just Don't Have a Bikini Body.'" *People.com*, October 9, 2015. https://people.com/style/drew-barrymore-i-am-who-i-am-and-i-just-dont-have-a-bikini-body/

43. Branch, K. "Jennifer Aniston on Bringing the #FreetheNipple Movement to the Masses First." *Vogue online*, August 10, 2017. https://www.vogue.com/article/jennifer-aniston-justin-theroux-aveeno-beauty-wellness-friends-hair-reese-witherspoon

44. "Kelly Clarkson Opens Up About the Darkest Time of Her Career." *Attitude online*, October 26, 2017. https://attitude.co.uk/article/kelly-clarkson-opens-up-about-the-darkest-time-in-her-career/16131/

45. Stern, A. and Mizoguchi, K. "Kelly Clarkson Says It's 'Really Crucial' to Instill Self-Esteem in Her Kids: 'Always Stand Up for Yourself.'" *People.com*, October 13, 2017. https://people.com/parents/kelly-clarkson-says-its-really-crucial-to-instill-self-esteem-in-her-kids-always-stand-up-for-yourself/

46. Edge, A. and Sands, N. "Katy Perry Opens Up About Being a Judge on American Idol: 'I'm a Straight Shooter.'" *People.com*, November 27, 2017.. https://people.com/music/katy-perry-american-idol-judge-straight-shooter/

47. Quinn, D. "Demi Lovato Reveals the Key to Surviving 'Bad Body Image Days.'" *People.com*, April 12, 2017. https://people.com/bodies/demi-lovato-key-to-surviving-bad-body-image-days/

48. "Serena Williams Sits Down with Common to Talk about Race and Identity." The Undefeated *online*, December 19, 2016. http://theundefeated.com/features/serena-williams-sits-down-with-common-to-talk-about-race-and-identity/

49. Winfrey, O. "What I Know for Sure." *Oprah.com*, 2018. http://www.oprah.com/omagazine/oprah-winfrey-on-body-image-what-i-know-for-sure-by-oprah

50. Kaufman, A. "I Had a Heart-to-Heart About Body Image with Amy Schumer." *LA Times online*, April 19, 2018. http://www.latimes.com/entertainment/movies/la-et-mn-amy-schumer-i-feel-pretty-20180419-story.html

51. Dawn, R. "Amy Schumer Opens Up about Body Image: 'I'm What Hollywood Calls Very Fat.'" *Today.com*, March 7, 2017. https://www.today.com/popculture/amy-schumer-opens-about-body-image-i-m-what-hollywood-t108941

52. Kaufman, A. "I Had a Heart-to-Heart About Body Image with Amy Schumer." *LA Times online,* April 19, 2018. http://www.latimes.com/entertainment/movies/la-et-mn-amy-schumer-i-feel-pretty-20180419-story.html

53. "Ashley Graham on Authenticity and Being a Body Image Activist." *Glamour online*, November 1, 2016. https://www.glamour.com/story/women-of-the-year-ashley-graham

54. "Ashley Graham on Authenticity and Being a Body Image Activist." *Glamour online*, November 1, 2016. https://www.glamour.com/story/women-of-the-year-ashley-graham

55. Graham, A. "Plus Size? More Like My Size." *TEDx Talks*, April, 2015. https://www.ted.com/talks/ashley_graham_plus_size_more_like_my_size?language=en

56. Graham, A. "Plus Size? More Like My Size." *TEDx Talks*, April, 2015. https://www.ted.com/talks/ashley_graham_plus_size_more_like_my_size?language=en

57. Price, L. "7 Times Jennifer Lawrence Got Candid About Body Image." *People.com*, April 8, 2016. https://people.com/celebrity/jennifer-lawrence-on-body-image/

58. Haiken, M. "Lady Gaga Puts Bulimia and Body Image on the Table in a Big Way." *Forbes online*, September 26, 2012.. https://www.forbes.com/sites/melaniehaiken/2012/09/26/lady-gaga-puts-bulimia-and-body-image-on-the-table-in-a-big-way/#64aa76342e14

59. "I Love Eating Pasta and Pizza": Lady Gaga Blames 25lb Weight Gain on Her Dad's Delicious Food. *Daily Mail online*, September 21, 2012. https://www.dailymail.co.uk/tvshowbiz/article-2206418/Lady-Gaga-blames-25lb-weight-gain-dads-delicious-food.html

60. Prakash, N. "Lady Gaga Has a Powerful Message for Her Super Bowl Shamers." *Glamour online*, February 8, 2017. https://www.glamour.com/story/lady-gaga-powerful-instagram-response-to-body-shamers

61. Hammel, S. "Tyra Banks: How I Talk to Girls honestly and Openly About Weight." *People.com*, May 9, 2014. https://people.com/bodies/tyra-banks-talks-weight-self-esteem-in-mentoring-girls-for-tzone-foundation/

62. Schnurr, S. "It's Been 10 Years Since Tyra Banks Told Everyone to 'Kiss My Fat Ass.'" *E-News online*. https://www.eonline.com/ca/news/826180/it-s-been-10-years-since-tyra-banks-told-everyone-to-kiss-my-fat-ass

63. Hammel, S. "Tyra Banks: How I Talk to Girls honestly and Openly About Weight." *People.com*, May 9, 2014. https://people.com/bodies/tyra-banks-talks-weight-self-esteem-in-mentoring-girls-for-tzone-foundation/

## ABOUT THE AUTHOR

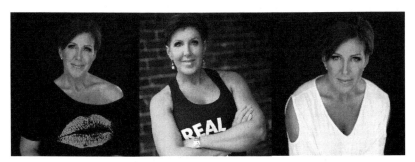

PHOTOGRAPHY CREDIT TO SKAZKA MAGES – WWW.SKAZKAIMAGES.COM

Lori Mork is an expert in the field of health and wellness, mindset, body positivity, and helping women create sustainable fitness. She is a fierce and dynamic author, speaker, former fitness champion, reformed dieting-junkie, and kick-ass coach to thousands of women worldwide.

With over twenty-seven years of experience in the fitness industry, Lori has witnessed firsthand the mass destruction of the female mind, body, and soul when unrealistic ideals and quick-fix lifestyles are forced down their throats by society, and now social media.

Having hit rock-bottom herself after decades of crazy fad diets, Lori found her way to freedom from society's impossible ideals and created balanced, long-term wellness on her own terms. Sharing this "piece of the puzzle," she now empowers her clients to reclaim control of how they feel about themselves.

When she isn't helping women reach their wellness goals or rock the shit out of their bodies, Lori spends her free time with her two children, her two dogs, and bottles of pinot grigio (#moderation). Lori's ultimate goal is to help women own our power and tell the haters or nay-sayers to "*Kiss My Curvy Assets!*"

**www.lorimork.com**
**ig: lori.mork | fb: lorimorkcoach | youtube: Lori Mork | tw: MorkLori**

## JOIN THE #KISSMYCURVYASSETS MOVEMENT

As women, when we stand together, have each other's backs, and show the world that we control our own body ideals and how we feel about ourselves, we can take over the world! **A CURVES AND ASSETS WORLD DOMINATION**!

The book gave you all the tools you need, so you can kick ass in the body rockin' department. Now, I need you to shout it from the rooftops!

- Share pictures of how you **ROCK THE SHIT OUT OF YOUR BODY!**

- Share your confidence, esteem, and badassery with all of us, and inspire others to come along on this exhilarating and empowering adventure.

- Share with us how you owned the shit you got, turned devastations into inspirations, and told any naysayers to **#KISSMYCURVYASSETS**

This is more than just a book... this is a movement of thousands, and hopefully millions, of women all over the world, so PLEASE SHARE YOUR HOT ASSETS and INSPIRING JOURNEY by using the below hashtag on social media:

### *#KISSMYCURVYASSETS*

I also want to hear your stories, so feel free to message me directly at **lori@lorlmork.com** or **www.lorimork.com**.

Hot AF women all over the world, I am talking to you, I want to see **YOU** rocking the shit out of your **body**!

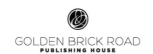

### GOLDEN BRICK ROAD
**PUBLISHING HOUSE**

## LOCKING ARMS AND HELPING EACH OTHER DOWN THEIR GOLDEN BRICK ROAD

At Golden Brick Road Publishing House, we lock arms with ambitious people and create success through a collaborative, supportive, and accountable environment. We are a boutique shop that caters to all stages of business around a book. We encourage women empowerment, and gender and cultural equality by publishing single author works from around the world, and creating in-house collaborative author projects for emerging and seasoned authors to join.

Our authors have a safe space to grow and diversify themselves within the genres of poetry, health, sociology, women's studies, business, and personal development. We help those who are natural born leaders, step out and shine! Even if they do not yet fully see it for themselves. We believe in empowering each individual who will then go and inspire an entire community. Our Director, Ky-Lee Hanson, calls this: "The Inspiration Trickle Effect"

If you want to be a public figure that is focused on helping people and providing value, but you do not want to embark on the journey alone, then we are the community for you.

To inquire about our collaborative writing opportunities or to bring your own idea into fruition, reach out to us at:

www.goldenbrickroad.pub

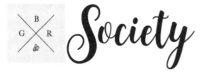

**Connect with our authors and readers at GBRSociety.com**

*Kiss My Curvy Assets* takes a blunt approach towards crushing body image stigmas and helps women embrace their badassery. This is not your average health, fitness, or wellness self-help book. It is witty, sassy, full on laugh-your-ass-off humor meets raw, empowering, tangible, results-driven coaching — all in one.

As a fitness and wellness coach with almost three decades of experience specializing in mindset and hormone health, Lori shows us:

- The calories you consume do not equal your self-worth

- Happiness and self-esteem play a huge role in achieving goals (more so than the bathroom scale or overtraining yourself)

- We should be embracing our unique assets instead of battling with, changing or transforming them

- You are hot AF regardless of what is happening on social media or within society

This book helps you to feel strong and healthy from the inside-out. Let's put down the waist trainers and magic fitness pixie dust! Girl, it is time to rock the sh!t out of your body - every curve and asset!

Join Lori on a journey of crushing internal demons, dispelling diet and fitness fads, smashing scales, and ending negative selftalk with your body. Learn to supercharge your hormone health and orgasms! Buckle up - it's gonna be an enlightening and exhilarating ride!